Praise for
My Lobotomy

"The lobotomy, although terrible, was not the greatest injury done to him. His greatest misfortune, as his own testimony makes clear, was being raised by parents who could not give him love. The lobotomy, he writes, made him feel like a Frankenstein monster. But that's not quite right. By the age of twelve, he already felt that way. It's this that makes *My Lobotomy* one of the saddest stories you'll ever read." —William Grimes, *New York Times*

"Dully's tale is a heartbreakingly sad story of a life seriously, tragically interrupted. All Howard Dully wanted was to be normal. His entire life has been a search for normality. He did what he had to do to survive. This book is his legacy, and it is a powerful one."
—*San Francisco Chronicle*

"In *My Lobotomy* Howard Dully tells more of the story that so many found gripping in a National Public Radio broadcast: how his stepmother joined with a doctor willing to slice into his brain with "ice picks" when he was all of twelve years old."
—*New York Daily News*

"[Dully's] memoir is vital and almost too disturbing to bear—a piece of recent history that reads like science fiction. . . . Dully, the only patient to ever request his file, speaks eloquently. It's a voice to crash a server, and to break your heart."
—*Cleveland Plain Dealer*

"The value of the book is in the indomitable spirit Dully displays throughout his grueling saga. . . . By coming to grips with his past and shining a light into the dark corners of his medical records, Dully shows that regardless of what happened to his brain, his heart and soul are ferociously strong."   *—Chicago-Sun Times*

"Compelling."   *—Washington Post*

"[A] plainspoken, heart-wrenching memoir."
                                                        —San Jose Mercury News

"Hard to put down."   *—The Record*

"Gut-wrenching . . . A profoundly disturbing survivor's tale."
                                                        —Kirkus Reviews

"A readable, well-crafted integration of Dully's own life and hospitalizations, and mental health conditions of the era. The book raises important issues about juvenile psychiatric treatment even today. Intense and moving."   *—Library Journal*

MY LOBOTOMY

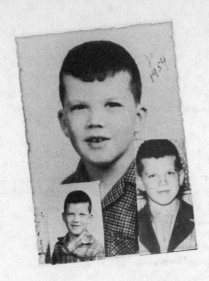

MY LOBOTOMY

— A Memoir —

HOWARD DULLY
and Charles Fleming

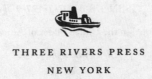

THREE RIVERS PRESS

NEW YORK

This is a true story. However, in the interest of protecting the privacy of certain individuals, some names and identities have been changed.

Published in the United States by Three Rivers Press, an imprint of the
Crown Publishing Group, a division of Random House, Inc., New York.
www.crownpublishing.com

Three Rivers Press and the Tugboat design are registered trademarks of
Random House, Inc.

Originally published in slightly different form in hardcover in the United States by
Crown Publishers, an imprint of the Crown Publishing Group,
a division of Random House, Inc., New York, in 2007.

The medical records used in this book are from the Walter Freeman and James Watts
Collections, Special Collections and University Archives, The Gelman Library,
The George Washington University.

Library of Congress Cataloging-in-Publication Data

Dully, Howard.
My Lobotomy / Howard Dully and Charles Fleming.—1st ed.
p. cm.
1. Dully, Howard, 1948– 2. Psychosurgery—Patients—United States—
Biography. 3. Frontal lobotomy—Patients—United States—
Biography. I. Fleming, Charles. II. Title.
[DNLM: 1. Personal Narratives. 2. Psychosurgery. 3. Patient.
WL 370 D883m 2007]
RD594.D85 2007
617.4'81—dc22 2007006070

ISBN 978-0-307-38127-9

Printed in the United States of America

Design by Lauren Dong

10 9 8 7 6 5 4 3 2 1

First Paperback Edition

To all of us, victims and survivors,
who keep going no matter what

Contents

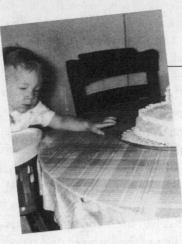

Preface

My name is Howard Dully. I'm a bus driver. I'm a husband, and a father, and a grandfather. I'm into doo-wop music, travel, and photography.

I'm also a survivor: In 1960, when I was twelve years old, I was given a transorbital, or "ice pick," lobotomy.

My stepmother arranged it. My father agreed to it. Dr. Walter Freeman, the father of the American lobotomy, told me he was going to do some "tests." It took ten minutes and cost two hundred dollars.

The surgery damaged me in many ways. But it didn't "fix" me, or turn me into a robot. So my family put me into an institution.

I spent the next four decades in and out of insane asylums, jails, and halfway houses. I was homeless, alcoholic, and drug-addicted. I was lost. I knew I wasn't crazy. But I knew something was wrong with me. Was it the lobotomy? Was it something else? I hadn't been a bad kid. I hadn't ever hurt anyone. Or had I? Was there something I had done, and forgotten—something so horrible that I deserved a lobotomy?

I asked myself that question for more than forty years. I thought about my lobotomy all the time, but I never talked about it. It was my terrible secret. What had been so *wrong* with me?

In 1998, when I was fifty, things changed. I had suffered a heart attack. I had married a woman I really loved. I had gotten clean and sober, and gone back to school and earned a degree. People who met me didn't know I'd had a lobotomy, or spent ten years in mental hospitals. They met a big man—I'm six foot seven and 330 pounds—with a big mustache and a big laugh whose job was driving special education kids to school on a yellow school bus.

They didn't see the man who was tormented by his shadowy past. Then Dr. Freeman died. My stepmother died. My dad and I had never talked about the past, and now he was in poor health, too. I was afraid all the people who really knew what had happened to me would be gone soon.

So I decided to try to find out what had been done to me. I sat down in front of my computer, logged on to the Internet, and typed in the words "Dr. Walter Freeman."

So began a journey that, four years later, brought me to Washington, D.C. I had met a pair of radio producers who were doing a program on lobotomy for NPR. They had arranged permission for me to see Dr. Walter Freeman's lobotomy archives. Even though Freeman personally lobotomized more than five thousand patients and paved the way for the lobotomies of tens of thousands more, I was the first one in history to show up asking to see his files.

The archivists handed me a manila folder. On the front of it were the words "DULLY, Howard."

The great mystery of my life was inside. The question that had haunted me for more than forty years was about to be answered.

MY LOBOTOMY

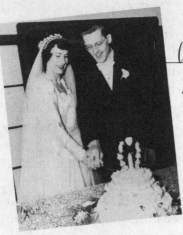

Chapter 1

June

This much I know for sure: I was born in Peralta Hospital in Oakland, California, on November 30, 1948. My parents were Rodney Lloyd Dully and June Louise Pierce Dully. I was their first child, and they named me Howard August Dully, after my father's father. Rodney was twenty-three. June was thirty-four.

They had been married less than a year. Their wedding was held on Sunday, December 28, 1947, three days after Christmas, at one o'clock in the afternoon, at the Westminster Presbyterian Church in Sacramento, California. The wedding photographs show an eager, nervous couple. He's in white tie and tails, with a white carnation in his lapel. She's in white satin, and a veil decorated with white flowers. They are both dark-haired and dark-eyed. Together they are cutting the cake—staring at the cake, not at each other—and smiling.

A reception followed at 917 Forty-fifth Street, at the home of my mother's uncle Ross and aunt Ruth Pierce. My father's mother attended. So did his two brothers. One of them, his younger brother, Kenneth, wore a tuxedo all the way up from San Jose on the train.

My father's relatives were railroad workers and lumberjack types from the area around Chehalis and Centralia, Washington. My dad spent his summers in a lumber camp with one of his uncles. They were logging people.

My father's father was an immigrant, born in 1899 in a place called Revel, Estonia, in what would later be the Soviet Union. When he left Estonia, his name was August Tulle. When he got to America, where he joined his brothers, Alexander and John—he had two sisters, Marja and Lovisa, who he left behind in Estonia—he was called August Dully. He later added the first name Howard, because it sounded American to him.

My father's mother was the child of immigrants from Ireland. She was born Beulah Belle Cowan in Litchfield, Michigan, in 1902. Her family later moved to Portland, Oregon, in time for Beulah to attend high school, where she was so smart she skipped two grades.

August went to Portland, too, because that's where his brothers were. According to his World War I draft registration card, he was brown-haired, blue-eyed, and of medium height. He got work as a window dresser for the Columbia River Ship Company. He became a mason. He met the redheaded Beulah at a dance. She told her mother that night, "I just met the man I'm going to marry." She was sixteen. A short while later, they tied the knot and took a freighter to San Francisco for their honeymoon, and stayed. A 1920 U.S. Census survey shows them living in an apartment building on Fourth Street. Howard A. Dully was now a naturalized citizen, working as a laborer in the shipyards.

Sometime after, they moved to Washington, where my grandfather went to work on the railroads. They started having sons—Eugene, Rodney, and Kenneth—before August got sick with tuberculosis. Beulah believed he caught it on that freighter going to San Francisco. He died at home, in bed, on New Year's Day, 1929. My dad was three years old. His baby brother was only fourteen months old.

Beulah Belle never remarried. She was hardheaded and strong-willed. She said, "I will never again have a man tell me what to do."

But she had a hard time taking care of her family. She couldn't keep up payments on the house. When she lost it, the boys went to stay with relatives. My dad was sent to live with an aunt and uncle at age six, and was shuffled from place to place after that. By his own account, he lived in six different cities before he finished high school—born in Centralia, Washington; then shipped around Oregon to Marshfield, Grants Pass, Medford, and Eugene; then to Ryderwood, Washington, where he and his brother Kenneth lived in a logging camp with their former housekeeper Evelyn Townsend and her husband, Orville Black.

At eighteen, Rod left Washington to serve with the U.S. Army, enlisting in San Francisco on December 9, 1943. Though he later was reluctant to talk about it, I know from my uncles that he was sent overseas and stationed in France. He served with the 723rd Railroad Division, laying track in an area near L'Aigle, France, that was surrounded by mines. One of my uncles told me that my father never recovered from the war. He said, "The man who went away to France never came back. He was damaged by what he saw there."

But another of my uncles told me Rod bragged about having a German girlfriend, so I guess it wasn't all bad. Not as bad as his brother Gene, who joined the army and got sent to Australia and New Guinea, where he developed malaria and tuberculosis and almost died. He weighed one hundred pounds when he came back to America, and lived at a military hospital in Livermore, California, for a long time after that.

By the time Rod finished his military service, his mother had left her job with Western Union Telegraph, in the Northwest, and moved to Oakland to work for the Southern Pacific Railroad. She was later made a night supervisor, working in the San Francisco office on Market Street. She would still be working there when I was born.

My mother's folks came from the other end of the economic spectrum. June was the daughter of Daisy Seulberger and Hubert O. Pierce—German on her mother's side, English on her father's. Daisy grew up wealthy, married Pierce, and had three children: Gordon, June, and Hugh. When Pierce died, Daisy married Delos Patrician, another wealthy Bay Area businessman. She moved her family to Oakland, into a huge, three-story shingled home on Newton Avenue. June spent her childhood there.

After his military service, my father relocated to the Bay Area and started taking classes at San Francisco Junior College, learning to be a teacher and doing his undergraduate work in elementary education.

Over the summers, he got part-time work at a popular high Sierras vacation spot, Tuolumne Meadows, in Yosemite. He met a young woman there, working as a housekeeper, who captured his eye. Her name was June.

She was tall, dark, and athletic, and for Rod she was a real catch. She was a graduate of the University of California at Berkeley, where she had been active with the Alpha Xi Delta sorority, and had a certificate to teach nursery school. She was from a well-known Oakland family, and for several years she had been a fixture on the local social scene. During the war she had worked in Washington, D.C., as a private secretary to the U.S. congressman from her district. When she returned to Oakland, she often had her name in the newspapers, hosting luncheons and teas for her society friends.

She had been courted by quite a few young men, but her controlling mother, Daisy, drove all the boyfriends away. When she met Rod, June was still beautiful, but she was no longer what you'd call young, especially not at that time. She was thirty-two. Being unmarried at that age during the 1940s was almost like being a spinster.

Their courtship was sudden and passionate. They fell in love over the summer of 1946, and saw each other in San Francisco and Berkeley through the next year. When June returned to work in Yosemite in the summer of '47, this time at Glen Aulin Camp, Rod left for the lumberyards of northern California and southern Oregon, where he was determined to make enough money to marry June in style. His letters over that summer were eager and filled with love. He was full of plans and promises—for his career, their wedding, the house he would buy her, the family they would have. He was worried that he was not the man June's mother wanted, or from the right level of society, but he was determined to prove himself. "I expect to make you happy. I won't marry you and take you into a life you won't be happy in," he wrote. "I'm happy now, much happier than I've ever been before in my life, cause you're my little dream girl and my dream is coming true."

After a hard summer of logging work, the plans for the wedding were made. The ceremony was held three days after Christmas in Sacramento. According to a newspaper story a week later, the couple was "honeymooning in Carmel" after a ceremony in which "the bride wore a white satin gown with a sweetheart neckline, long sleeves ending in points at the wrists and full skirt with a double peplum pointed at the front. Her full-length veil of silk net was attached to a bandeau of seed pearls and orange blossoms. She also carried a handkerchief which has been in her family for 75 years."

The bride was given away by her uncle Ross, in whose Sacramento house she had been living. The groom's best man was his brother Kenneth.

According to family stories, some of June's family objected. Rod was too young for June, Daisy said, and didn't have good prospects. June may have been uncomfortable with the relative poverty she was marrying into, too. My dad later told people that he got into a fender bender not long after he met June, and that his feelings were hurt when she said she was embarrassed to be seen driving around in his banged-up car.

With a wife to support, my father left school. He and my mother moved up north, to Medford, Oregon, where Rod returned to the lumber business and went to work as a lumber tallyman with the Southern Oregon Sugar Pine Corporation in Central Point, two miles outside of Medford.

Soon the young married couple had a baby on the way—me. Near the end of her term, my mother left my dad in Medford and moved in with her mother in Oakland, a pattern she would repeat for the births of all her children.

If everything had gone as planned, she probably would have returned to Medford and raised a family.

But my father had some bad luck. One morning on a work break he became incoherent and had to be taken by ambulance to a Medford hospital. He was treated for sun stroke and sent back to work. When his symptoms returned, he saw another doctor and was treated for heat stroke. When he still did not improve, Rod left Medford and went to live with June's family in the big house in Oakland. He recovered but was told not to resume any kind of hard, physical outdoor work. The lumber business was over for him. He would never return to the Northwest.

I was carried to full term, according to the birth records, and I was a normal, healthy child, delivered early in the morning by a doctor named John Henry. I was a big baby—nine pounds and twenty-four inches long. (I come by that naturally. My parents were both big. My mother was six feet and my father was six feet three inches. My younger brother, Brian, is six feet ten inches.) Photographs of me when I was a baby show a big, goofy-looking infant with bright eyes and a healthy appetite. In one picture I am reaching out for a slice of cake. My father says I was a cheerful, happy, friendly baby who was doted upon by his mother.

They gave me my grandfather's adopted American name— Howard August Dully. To this day my uncle Kenneth says I'm the one Dully who looks most like him.

My father's occupation was listed on my birth certificate as "Talley man, Southern Sugar Pine Lumber Co., Medford, Ore." But he never went back to that job. After my birth, he moved his new family into a one-bedroom apartment at Spartan Village, a low-income student-housing complex near San Jose State University. He got a sales job at San Jose Lumber, a lumberyard right down the street from our apartment, and resumed his studies at the university.

I have very few memories of living at Spartan Village. The clearest one is a memory of fear. There was a playground there and my dad built me a choo-choo train out of fifty-gallon oil drums and lumber. I was proud of it, and proud that my dad had built it.

But there was a big, open field of weeds next to the apartment complex. I was afraid of that field. I was afraid of what was in those weeds. There was a low place in the center of the field that kids would run into and disappear. I was afraid they wouldn't come out. I knew that if I went into that field I would fall in and not be able to come out. It's the first thing in my life I remember being afraid of.

In August 1951, when I was two and a half years old, Rodney and June had another son. They named him Brian. Like me, he was born healthy. I now had a roommate in our Spartan Village apartment.

In some families, the arrival of the second son is the end of the world for the first son, because now he has to share his mother with a stranger. Not in my family. My dad said Brian's birth did not have any impact on my close relationship with June. *He* was responsible for Brian, while she concentrated all her love on me. "I was the one taking care of Brian," he said. "All she cared about was little Howard."

My father told me later that I was the most important person in my mother's life—more important, even, than him. I was the number-one son. "I could've dropped dead and it wouldn't have made a bit of difference," my dad said. "She had you."

When he completed his degree, my father was hired as an elementary school teacher in a one-room schoolhouse in a little town called Pollock Pines in the Sierras, about halfway between Sacramento and Lake Tahoe.

Most of my early childhood memories come from this place. Our house sat on a hill that sloped down to a bend in Highway 50, the two-lane road that led from Sacramento to Lake Tahoe. We had a little cocker spaniel named Blackie. He was hit by a car on that road, and killed, when I was about two years old.

I also remember sitting in a coffee shop in Placerville, having a soda with my mother. We were waiting for my father. Music was playing.

My mother's uncle Ross and aunt Ruth had a huge mountain cabin, so big it was more like a hunting lodge, farther up Highway 50, near a famous old resort called Little Norway. It had been built by my great-grandfather—Grandma Daisy's father—in the 1930s. The main building, which was two stories and filled with moose heads, was surrounded by pine trees and smaller cabins that were so primitive they had dirt floors. We used to stay in one of them when I was little.

In the winter, the snow was so deep we cut steps in it and climbed onto the cabin roof. Later on I learned to ski there, but my earliest memories of the snow are unhappy ones. I stepped into a snow drift that was so deep I sank in up to my waist and couldn't get out. This frightened me. I thought some kind of snow monster was going to come and eat me, and I began to cry.

My father thought it was the funniest thing he'd ever seen. I was terrified, but he was laughing. That made me mad at him.

I think I was a happy child. I remember walking the two blocks from our apartment to my father's work every day, my mother carrying the sack lunch she'd made for him. But I also remember not liking the way my mother made me dress. I had to wear colored shirts, and those little shorts that have straps to hold them up. They looked like those German lederhosen. Even as a kid I thought they were lame. I probably wanted to wear blue jeans.

My mother liked being a mother and she took naturally to it. In my favorite picture of her from that time, she's wearing a cap-sleeve shirt, a wide black belt, and a billowing skirt, and she's standing under a clothesline in the Spartan Village yard. She looks like she's calling to me, and she looks happy.

Family members have told me that she enjoyed life and laughed a lot. She wasn't serious, like my dad. She was more carefree, and liked to have fun.

In my memory, she was a very loving and indulgent mother. I remember being held and hugged and kissed by her. I remember being loved. I have fleeting pictures in my head of green grass, of sunshine, of running past my mother's full skirts. I remember her laughing.

My father was restless and ambitious. His desire for a better job moved us again. He left the one-room schoolhouse where he had been teaching in Pollock Pines and got another elementary school job in the nearby Camino school district.

He later took a job where his brother Kenneth was working, in the Barron Gray Cannery in San Jose, packing pineapple and other fruit for Dole. We moved in with Kenneth and his wife, Twila, and their four children in Saratoga, a San Jose suburb. This lasted until my mother got pregnant again.

Just like she did when she was pregnant with me and with Brian, she went to live with her mother for the last few months of her pregnancy. My dad stayed in Saratoga with me and Brian, crowded into his brother's house, while everyone waited for the baby to arrive.

Then he was born, and it was very bad. He was brain-damaged—so severely that the doctors said he was not expected to survive. The doctors said he had only half a brain. His name was Bruce. He was born in Oakland, in the Highland-Alameda County Hospital, and he stayed there.

But so did my mother. Something was wrong with her, too, and it was serious. The doctors had missed it. Maybe the symptoms had been covered up by the problems with her pregnancy. Maybe the doctors were so concerned about what was wrong with the baby that they didn't notice something was wrong with her. Maybe, like my father insisted later, it was because her family was too cheap to get her to a good private hospital.

Whatever the reason, by the time they figured out she was sick, it was too late for them to help her.

My mother died in the hospital twelve days after Bruce was born. Not until an autopsy was performed did her doctors realize she had cancer of the colon. According to her death certificate, the cause of death was "peritonitis, acute," brought on by a perforated colon, which was caused by colon cancer. The doctor's notes say she had been suffering from the cancer for months, but her death had followed the perforation of the colon by a matter of hours.

That is why my father almost did not see his wife before she died. It took a full day for someone from Daisy's family to call him at work and let him know there was a problem. When he finally arrived at the hospital, he had to meet with a doctor before he could see his wife. Someone from Daisy's family—her brother Gordon, my father said—had told the doctors that June and Rod were separated, and that he wasn't really part of the family anymore. My father had to convince the doctors this wasn't true before they would let him in.

By the time he got to see her, my mother was in a coma. Her eyes were open, but she was incoherent. She died that night. She was thirty-nine.

The autopsy was conducted the following day. Her own physician participated. He hadn't known anything about the disease that killed her until after she was dead. Some family members would remember later that she had complained to her doctor repeatedly that she didn't feel well, that she had pains. The doctor had chalked it up to morning sickness, and paid no attention to it.

My mother died without ever leaving the Oakland county hospital, without ever saying good-bye to her two sons, and maybe without ever saying hello to her newborn. I don't know if she ever even laid eyes on Bruce.

Years later, I learned that she was cremated, and that her ashes were interred in the Chapel of Memories cemetery in Oakland. My father told me that the funeral service was attended by dozens of June's personal friends, by my father's mother and two brothers, and by June's two brothers—but not by her mother.

I don't know if my parents' marriage was a happy one. My dad always said it was. I have no reason to think it wasn't. But I learned many years later that one of the very last things my mother did in her life was change my name. I became, legally, Howard August *Pierce* Dully, taking on her maiden name as my second middle name. My father's mother told me my dad was very angry about this. June had done it without his permission.

Why? What difference would it make? Why did she care if Pierce was part of my name?

I never found out. But I did learn, years later, that after June's death her mother, Daisy, and brother Gordon tried to have me and Brian taken away from my father. Daisy filed papers to have me adopted by Gordon, so he could take us away from our dad and raise us as his own.

"Gordon wanted to adopt the kids" my dad told me later. "*He* would raise them, himself. He said I was a lousy father, that June should never have married me. If I'd had a gun, I would have shot him."

I wasn't conscious of any of this at the time. All I knew was I missed my mother, and she was gone. No one told me she was dead. I didn't understand that she was dead. But I understood that she was gone. My father told me so. One evening sometime after my mother's death, he told me she wasn't coming home.

It was almost dark. We were alone in the car. We were in San Jose, riding down Seventh Street in my dad's Plymouth station wagon. He told me my mother had gone away. She wasn't coming back. I wasn't ever going to see her again.

I was four years old, and I got very, very upset. I threw a terrible tantrum. I screamed and yelled. I needed to see my mother. I cried my eyes out and shouted that I wanted to see my mother. I *demanded* to see my mother.

It might have been better if he had just told me she was dead. Then I would have understood, maybe, what was going on. As it was, I thought she had left me. I was afraid she didn't want to see me. I was afraid she didn't love me.

What other explanation could there be? Why else would your mother leave you and never come back again, except that she didn't love you?

This was too painful for me. So I decided she was still there, somehow. I thought she could see me. She knew what I was doing. She was nearby, somewhere, smiling down at me, or crying, about what she saw me doing. I wasn't alone, even when I felt alone, because she was watching me.

I didn't tell anyone that I felt this way, or had these ideas. Maybe I knew it was all imagination, or maybe I was afraid they would tell me it wasn't true. I kept it to myself.

This was a very hard time for me. And I see now how hard it must have been for my father. He was twenty-seven years old. His wife—the woman he loved, the mother of his children—was dead. He himself had already suffered a stroke. He had two sons at home under the age of five, and a third son, severely retarded, who was probably going to die but who would require permanent professional care if he didn't. He was estranged from his in-laws, who had money—and who had conspired to take his sons away from him—and his own family had no money to speak of. And he didn't even have his own place. He was staying with his brother, living off the charity of his family. It must have been hard for that kind of man, born and raised like he was, to live like that.

For a few months after my mother's death we continued to live with my uncle Kenneth. We had to. My dad had started a new career. He had just gotten a new job, teaching elementary school in Los Altos.

Most people who know San Jose these days think of it as the center of the Silicon Valley, or as a bedroom community for the wealthier city of San Francisco—in either case, a place where rich people live. It's the oldest city in California—it was founded in 1777—and it was once the capital city of the original Spanish colony of Nueva California. For a while its primary business was supplying farms and canneries to feed San Francisco. Later on it would be a big military center. But when I was a kid, it was just another working-class town.

There was always money around San Jose, but most of it didn't live there. Even if they worked or owned businesses in San Jose, most of the people with money went home at night to places like Palo Alto, home of Stanford University, and ritzy communities like Mountain View, Saratoga, and Los Altos. Especially Los Altos, where rich people lived in big houses and drove expensive automobiles. These were people who played golf and rode horses. They didn't live in low-income housing for married students or have to move their families into their brothers' homes because they didn't have anyone to watch their kids.

Even though it was only ten miles away from my uncle Kenneth's house, Los Altos was like a different world. That's where my dad went to work every day. He had started teaching fifth grade at Hillview Elementary. Los Altos is where he spent his days before coming home at night to share the crowded house with his brother Kenneth.

It wasn't perfect, but pretty soon we lost that, too. My aunt Twila couldn't take the overcrowding. Kenneth told his brother that we had to go. My dad, who had spent his own childhood bouncing from place to place, had to find a new home for us, again.

My father's mother, my grandmother Beulah, was still living in San Francisco and working in the Southern Pacific offices on Market Street. To help us out, she moved down to Palo Alto and rented a little house—a kind of factory worker's house, with two bedrooms, a small kitchen, and a small living room—from a local Christian Scientist woman, and we all moved in together.

Beulah was a short, stout, tough Irish redhead who was very cosmopolitan and stylish, and extremely direct. Because Beulah was a strange name to us, we called her Grandma Boo. She was a working woman, and she had no time for nonsense. She ran a strict household, and, like my dad, she wasn't what you would call affectionate. Every afternoon she'd walk down to the train station and take the train north to work. Early the next morning she'd come back.

Because she worked and my father worked, someone had to come in and take care of the children. So my dad found a neighbor who would watch me and Brian during the day. She served us sugar-and-cinnamon toast. I remember the toast, I think, because I remember being hungry. I remember thinking about food a lot, and I remember searching for it in that house.

It was a dark, crowded place, with Grandma Boo's things and our things piled up everywhere. There was one bedroom for me and Brian at the front of the house, and one bedroom for my dad and Boo in the back. It had a curtain running down the middle of it, so they could each have some privacy. Hidden away in a corner of the room was a big cookie tin where Boo kept these delicious, soft oatmeal cookies.

I was *crazy* for those oatmeal cookies. I'd sneak down the hall and open the tin—while my dad and my grandmother were right there in the room, sleeping—and steal a couple of cookies. And not just once or twice, either. I made a career out of stealing those cookies.

We lived that way with Grandma Boo for about a year. I got old enough to start kindergarten. I remember being afraid to go. The school seemed like a big, scary place. I was afraid I'd get hurt there, or I'd get lost, or I wouldn't be able to find my way home.

It wasn't just the school. I was scared of a lot of things. I was afraid there were crocodiles under my bed at night. Later, when we moved again and I had to take the bus to school, I was afraid of that, too. I was so afraid that I'd get on the wrong bus, or get off at the wrong school. Things like that really terrified me.

Maybe it was because of my mother's death, but I was afraid a lot of the time. I remember having terrible nightmares.

One of them stayed with me into adulthood. In this dream, I am walking on a deserted city street. It's cold, and the city is gray. A long white car pulls slowly to the curb, and the door opens. I can't see who's inside, but I know they have come to get me. Then a rope, its end tied into a noose, comes out of the car and begins to slither along the sidewalk toward me. I know it's going to catch me and pull me in. I know I can't escape. I'm terrified and I want to run away, but I can't. I can't escape.

I always wake up before I find out who's in the car, or where they're taking me.

Other than the night terrors, I think I was a pretty normal kid. I was physical. I liked playing games. I had a mechanical mind. I would spend hours underneath the kitchen sink, pulling out all the pots and pans and trying to figure out how to stack them so they'd fit under there again. My father used to bring home things like broken radio sets for me to play with. I'd pull them apart and try to put them back together. My father always told people how impressed he was that I could put them back the right way—always figuring which tube went where, even though I was so little.

I don't remember whether I ever wondered what had happened to Bruce. To this day, I'm not sure where he was living at that time. I know that he surprised the doctors who delivered him and did not die as an infant. At some point he was able to leave the hospital. I found out later that my dad had found a Christian Science woman to look after him. But at the time his existence was all wrapped up in my mother's death. We never, ever talked about him.

In the end, my dad's new teaching job saved us from our cramped living arrangement with Grandma Boo. The families of Los Altos and the parents of my father's students at Hillview Elementary heard about my mother's death, and they came to our rescue. We started getting invitations to dinner. Me and Brian and my dad went to dinner at a bunch of people's houses. They fed us and clucked over us and made sure we were doing all right. They helped my dad with things like sewing and washing.

One of the women was especially helpful. She started doing laundry for us. Then she offered to babysit me and Brian. Her name was Lucille, but everyone called her Lou.

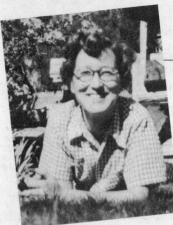

Chapter 2

Lou

My mother was a tall, handsome woman with strong features, wavy black hair, and a very feminine sense of fashion. In all of the pictures I have of her, she's dressed like she's going someplace special. She's wearing dresses, or nice skirts and blouses. She has her hair done nicely and she's wearing makeup. She looks pretty, and she looks like she looks that way on purpose. She's spent some time making herself beautiful.

Lou was the opposite. She was shorter, and plainer, and kind of mannish. She wore her curly hair cut short. She hardly ever wore makeup. In the pictures I have of her, she's dressed like she's going to work in the yard. She wore jeans, or pants, or slacks, but hardly ever skirts or dresses—which was unusual for that time—and checked shirts, like a farm woman. She was slender, and had a sort of girlish figure, but her presentation was more masculine than feminine. She wore round tortoiseshell glasses. She smoked non-filter cigarettes. She was all business.

Her full name was Shirley Lucille Hardin. She was the daughter of Herbert Sidney Hardin and Shirley Lucille Jackson, who was in turn the daughter of George William Gresley-Jackson and Shirley Lucille Daughterman. Lou was born in San Francisco—just like her mother and grandmother before her.

Her childhood was very unstable. Lou was born in 1919. Her

mother was born in 1900. So her mother was a just teenager when she had Lou. According to family stories, her mother was a real 1920s flapper, who bobbed her hair and danced the Charleston.

Lou's parents didn't have any interest in raising a child. Herbert seems to have disappeared right after her birth. Her mother then turned Lou over to the care of her own mother. She was raised by this grandmother, a widow whose husband passed away when Lou was a little girl.

Lou's mother went on to have at least four husbands. With one of them she had another daughter, named Virginia, a few years after Lou was born. Lou's father, Herbert, remarried a woman named Daphne, who was known as Nana, and spent most of his life in Idaho. He was an alcoholic, and worked as a house painter. After he retired, he moved back to the San Jose area, where he and Nana became good friends with Shirley and her new husband, Lynn Swindell. One of my cousins remembers them all getting together for bridge games.

So Lou, like my dad, didn't have a normal childhood, surrounded by good, traditional role models for healthy parenting.

Lou grew up around San Francisco. She had moved to the San Jose area by the time she was a teenager, and was going to Mountain View High School when she met her first husband. His name was Red Cox. He was a teenage runaway from Alabama. Red and Lou waited until they both graduated—and until Lou's grandmother had died—to get married. That same year, her mother married her fourth and last husband. By then, Lou's mother had moved to the San Jose area, too. For the first time in her life, Lou had a relationship with her real mother.

Lou and Red had two sons, Cleon and George. But she didn't take naturally to motherhood—at least not according to her niece, Linda Pickering, who as a little girl spent a lot of time around Lou. Linda remembered watching Lou raising George. When he was a little baby he would sit in his bassinet and cry. Finally Linda's mother would say, "Lou, that boy is hungry. Why don't you feed him?" Lou would say, "I just fed him. He isn't due to eat again for another hour." Then Linda's dad would say, "You better feed that baby, or else get him a watch."

"Because of the way she grew up," Linda said, "nobody ever taught her how to be a mother."

By the time she met my father, Lou was already divorced and was living with Cleon and George in the house in Los Altos that she'd shared with Red.

I don't remember meeting her. I don't remember her babysitting us, or doing our laundry, even though that's what I was told later. All I knew is one day she wasn't there, and the next day she was. My father said later that he had known her for about a year and a half before he proposed and she accepted. Soon enough, we all moved in together.

That would have been about 1955, when I was seven. *Rebel Without a Cause* and *Blackboard Jungle* were hits at the movies, which meant that rock 'n' roll and the American teenager were both officially on the map. On TV, there was *I Love Lucy* and *Dragnet* and *The Honeymooners*. Bill Haley's "Rock Around the Clock" was playing on the radio. It was a cool time to be a young person. It seemed like the whole country was changing.

Compared to us, Lou and her ex-husband seemed rich. His full name was Cleon Morgan Cox II, which sounds like a rich guy's name. He was a contractor who sometimes worked as a carpenter. He'd been married to Lou for fourteen years before they divorced. The family gossip said that he was a drunk.

The house they'd lived in, at 376 Hawthorne in Los Altos, was a nice, modest, ranch-style place, white and yellow, with a big pepper tree in the backyard and a couple of pine trees, and bordered by an old-fashioned split-rail redwood fence in the front. Red Cox had bought it in 1953. It was on a quiet, shady street a few blocks away from Hillview Elementary, where my dad taught and where I would go to school. It was about three-quarters of a mile from the little stretch of "downtown" Los Altos.

With all of us living in it together, the two-bedroom house on

Hawthorne was crowded. The four boys—me and Brian, Cleon and George—shared a single bedroom outfitted with two sets of bunk beds. My dad and Lou had the other bedroom, down a hallway that was "restricted." We were not allowed to go down there, into their hallway, their bathroom, or their bedroom.

The house was cramped, but it was fun. I liked having stepbrothers. Cleon, who was known as Binky, was about five years older than me, but George was just a few months older than me. I liked having a kid around who was my own age. George and I spent a lot of time playing outside, in a sandbox behind the house, or climbing that big pepper tree. My father liked to barbecue, so we had cookouts whenever the weather was warm enough.

My father also liked to build things. He always had a project going. He'd pick up lumber from the street, or from construction sites, and store it at home. One summer he built a homemade swimming pool in the front yard. He had bought these army surplus tents, made of heavy canvas, and figured out a way to stitch them together. Then he built a kind of platform around them, and filled the stitched-together tents with water.

It was leaky, and it was messy, and it was kind of funky, but it was a swimming pool. That was terrific. I have pictures of me and George and Brian, suntanned and wet, splashing around and having a great time. We had swimming races, competing to see who could run and jump in and swim the most circles around the pool without coming up for air. There's even a picture of Grandma Boo getting into the act, standing in this funny homemade swimming pool wearing a flowered bathing suit and a bathing cap, smiling into the camera.

To solve the overcrowding problem, my dad also built an addition to the back of the house on Hawthorne. That became Cleon's bedroom, so it was just me and Brian and George sharing a room.

Leaving the cramped house with Grandma Boo for a new house with a new mom and new stepbrothers was a big change. So was moving from San Jose to Los Altos. Socially, that was a giant change.

I already knew about Los Altos. Everybody knew about Los Altos. It was like the Beverly Hills of San Jose. It was an uptight, upper-middle-class, or even upper-class, community. This was where the doctors and lawyers lived, where the wealthy people lived. The houses in Los Altos were larger and statelier than anyplace I'd ever lived, and you never saw so many Lincolns and Cadillacs, and foreign cars. It seemed exotic. It was green and leafy. The roads were lined with redwood trees, pepper trees, and oaks. The sidewalks and backyards were shaded by fruit trees, too. I especially liked apricots. You could pick your lunch on the way to school and eat your fill.

The little strip of downtown was like something out of a storybook. The main drag was filled with attractive little shops. There was a five-and-dime store in the center of the block called Sprouse Ritz. The supermarket where we did our grocery shopping, Whitecliff Market, was just around the corner. Down the street was Clint's, an ice cream parlor with a giant ice cream cone on the roof. At the end of that block was a quaint one-story shopping center, where the buildings were all made of dark-stained redwood. The parking lot was always full of nice-looking cars—especially those wood-paneled station wagons that rich suburban housewives used to drive.

We could never have afforded to live there on our own. I'm not sure my dad could have afforded to own his own home even in San Jose. For sure he couldn't have bought a house in Los Altos, not on an elementary school teacher's salary. (My dad told me he was hired there at a starting salary of $4,000 per year.) So it must have been the fact that Lou already owned the house on Hawthorne that made it possible for us to live in Los Altos.

This might have grated on my dad. He was a proud man, and this was the 1950s. Women weren't supposed to be the breadwinners, and they weren't supposed to hold the purse strings, or the deed to the ranch.

It also might have given my dad an extra reason to work extra hard. Because he started working very hard. Every day he went to teach at Hillview, just like he had been doing. But now that he was a two-family man he took a second job working as a motion-picture processor on the swing shift at an Eastman Kodak production facility in Palo Alto. He'd come home from teaching, eat something, then change his clothes and go out again. He'd work from six to midnight, when the graveyard shift started, then he'd come home and sleep and get up and teach again.

But that wasn't enough. I don't know if he needed extra money, or felt he needed to pull his own weight, or just wanted a reason to be out of the crowded house and away from all those kids. Whatever it was, he took a third job. He started working on weekday afternoons and all day Saturday and Sunday as a checker at Whitecliff Market. During the week, he'd leave school, go to Whitecliff, work a few hours, come home and grab a quick bite, then go to Kodak for his swing shift.

That wasn't enough, either. He got a *fourth* job. He signed on as a crossing guard, before school and after school. He'd leave the house early in the morning and stand out there with another Hillview teacher, raising and lowering this big sign so the kids could get across the street. He'd leave school and do it again after classes ended, then go to Whitecliff, then come home to change, then go to Eastman Kodak.

I'm not sure how long he did that, but after a while that still wasn't enough. He enlisted in the National Guard, and began taking military classes and undergoing training on the weekends.

The obsession with work was a lifelong thing with my dad. My uncle Kenny told me that when he and my dad were in high school, and living in that logging camp in Ryderwood, Washington, my dad was the same way. There were fifty kids in their high school, and there were three part-time jobs available for the high school boys. "Rod had all three of them," Kenny said. "He was the janitor, he swept up in the pool hall, and he worked in the meat market at the company store."

Somehow he also found time to continue his education, too. He studied part-time at Stanford on the nights he wasn't working and on the weekends that he wasn't doing his National Guard service.

We didn't see much of him. When he was home at all, he'd come in tired and sit down in front of the TV with a beer and a little snack and fall straight to sleep. Me and the other kids got yelled at if we made noise. Dad's sleep was the most important thing, whether he was taking a nap in his room or snoring in his easy chair. We'd get in real trouble if we woke him up.

I got in trouble all the time.

Lou was a stern stepmother, and she ran a tight ship. She kept a clean house. I've never lived in such a clean house. I *liked* living in a clean house, but with Lou it was a kind of mania.

For example, not long after we moved in with her, she started inspecting and then wiping my butt. She'd make me take down my pants and underpants, and bend me over. If she didn't like what she saw, she'd take a washcloth and wipe me—while complaining about how dirty I was.

She did this with my brother Brian, too. And maybe with him it made sense. He was old enough to wipe himself, but he was only four, and he hadn't had a mother around for most of his life, so maybe he wasn't doing such a good job of it. But I was seven years old! I didn't need anyone to wipe my butt. It was traumatic for me. It was humiliating to have someone make me bend over and take my pants down. I hated it.

Lou was a good cook. She made pork chops with mashed potatoes and homemade gravy. She baked turkeys, and roast beef, and she cooked liver. She was big on salads and vegetables, which I didn't like at all. She made cornbread and homemade soups. I never knew her to use anything canned or powdered or packaged. She made good homemade cakes, even though I didn't like the way she did her icing—it wasn't that creamy, gooey kind that I liked. One of her famous dishes was Italian Delight. She'd take whatever was left over in the fridge and put it together with Italian sauce and spices and serve it over spaghetti. This was Lou's Friday night special.

But she was also very strict. She had rules about everything—you'd better do this, and you'd better *not* do that—and she always knew if you broke them. She could tell, even if you were at the other end of the house, whether you'd washed your hands before dinner. If you hadn't, you might get sent to your room.

You could get punished for yelling, for fighting, for coming home late from school, for not doing your homework, for losing your homework, for getting your school clothes dirty, for talking back, for not having proper table manners, and for any number of other things. Lou made everyone say "yes, ma'am" and "no, ma'am." She made everyone say "please" and "thank you." If you forgot, you got in trouble for that, too.

If you didn't behave, you either got sent to your room or you got spanked. Being sent to your room wasn't so bad. I didn't like being left out of the games, or being separated from my brothers, but I could do things in my room with my imagination. I could invent things. I had plastic cowboys and Indians, and army men, and I could make up stuff by myself.

The problem was the house was so small and cramped. If it was nighttime or a rainy day, and the other boys weren't playing outside, I couldn't be punished by being sent to my room—because we all shared a room. So, a lot of the time, I got spanked.

To be honest, I deserved some kind of punishment. I was a troublemaker. I'd get restless or bored, and I'd start to misbehave.

For example, I liked scaring people. I would hide behind a door or behind the sofa and wait for someone to walk into the room. Then, when they were real close, I'd jump out and scream. I *loved* getting a reaction. Mostly I did it to George or Brian. Especially Brian.

I also liked to attack Brian, or attack his stuff. I'd watch him carefully build a castle out of blocks. I'd watch him make the walls and the tower, and maybe put a bridge over his imaginary moat. I'd wait until he had everything perfect. Then I'd come swooping down like an invading horde. I was Attila the Hun. I was Genghis Khan. I'd descend on his unprotected castle and demolish it. I thought this was the funniest thing in the world. I'd storm in, attack him, and then storm out again, laughing my head off while he cried about his ruined castle.

It never occurred to me that I was hurting him, or even upsetting him. I just thought the idea of it was so hysterical. That moment of surprise was so much fun that I never really thought about how it felt to be on the other end of it. So I got in trouble.

I also got in trouble at Lou's house for eating when I wasn't supposed to eat. She was very strict about food, just like she was strict about all the rules in that house. Meals were for mealtime. There was no snacking. If you were hungry, you went hungry and you waited until dinner.

I couldn't wait. I was a big kid. I was growing fast. I was hungry all the time. So I'd go into the kitchen and grab something to eat. Usually it was fruit. I particularly liked bananas. I'd take the banana and go up to my room and eat it there.

It wasn't just at home. I was hungry everywhere I went, and I learned to sneak or steal food. In the first grade at Hillview Elementary, I got caught committing my very first crime. I was hungry, as usual, and I was alone in the cloakroom, and I realized I was surrounded by other kids' lunch boxes. So I opened one and found some cherries and started chowing down. I got caught red-handed—literally, with cherry juice still on my fingers—and was punished. When I got home and told Lou what had happened, I got punished again, with a spanking.

Sometimes I got punished for things I shouldn't have been punished for at all. For example, I got punished for taking those bananas. Like I said, Lou ran a tight ship. If a banana was missing, she'd know it. I don't think she actually counted the bananas, but there was the problem of getting rid of the evidence. You couldn't hide a banana peel from her. She kept such a clean house that she'd find it no matter where you put it—in the trash, under the bed, wherever—and you'd get punished for stealing a banana. Imagine spanking a kid for taking food from his own house when he was hungry. But that's what happened, more times than I can remember.

So, between one thing and another, I got spanked a *lot*. When I was little, this was usually a pants-down, over-the-knee spanking. Lou would deliver some pretty sharp smacks, with her hand or with a wooden spoon, and give me a lecture. It was painful, and it was embarrassing.

With my dad, it was much more serious. When it was his turn to do the spanking, he didn't fool around. After he'd come home from work, Lou would take him aside and tell him what I had done. Sometimes she told him the truth. Sometimes she exaggerated or made things up. Sometimes she'd blame me for things the other boys did. Either way, my dad would punish me for it. He never asked me if it was true. He never asked me for my side of the story. He'd just say, "Howard!" and then take me outside.

With my dad, I got spanked with a piece of wood. I had to choose the piece of wood myself. This was tricky. If I chose a thick piece, it was going to hurt. But if I chose a thin piece and it broke, he'd finish the job with his hand, and that never broke. So I'd try to choose one in the middle, a board that would bend a little when he hit me but not break.

I got pretty good at choosing boards, because I got a lot of practice. I'm not sure what I did to deserve it, but I swear I remember some weeks when I got spanked every single day—either by Lou or by my father. I remember afternoons when Lou would say, "That's it. I'm telling your father when he gets home." I'd spend the rest of the day worrying about that, wondering what time he was going to get home and how badly I was going to get spanked when he did. I guess I was scared of him. He was a big man, and he was rough with me. He never really hurt me—like, to the point of putting me in the hospital—but I was afraid that one day he was going to.

Sometimes, in addition to the spanking, Lou would take something away—a toy, or a ball, or my bike. But the big punishment during that time, when we lived in the house on Hawthorne, was losing television privileges.

This was the 1950s. Television was a pretty new thing. There wasn't much of anything special on TV for kids, except maybe

Saturday morning cartoons. There was some boxing, and some roller derby, but that didn't interest me. There were lots of family shows. There was *Life of Riley* and *Bachelor Father*. But I didn't care about those too much, either. They weren't really made for children, and those families sure didn't look like *my* family.

But television did have *Disneyland*. Every Wednesday night there was *Disneyland*. This was the TV show hosted by Walt Disney—the name would later be changed to *Walt Disney Presents* and then to *Walt Disney's Wonderful World of Color*—and it was the biggest event of the week. I practically dreamed about watching *Disneyland*. I looked forward to it the way some kids look forward to Christmas.

If the boys had been good all week, we were all allowed to sit in front of the TV and watch the whole show. If we'd been *real* good, we were given a candy bar to eat while we watched.

For me, this was heaven—sitting in front of the TV, eating a candy bar, watching *Disneyland*. It didn't get any better than that. So taking these things away from me was the most effective punishment that Lou could think of. If I had been bad, the other boys would get a candy bar and I wouldn't. If I had been really bad, my punishment was not being allowed to watch *Disneyland* at all. I'd be sent to my room instead—still hungry, and with no candy bar—where I could hear Brer Rabbit singing "Everybody's Got a Laughing Place" or Fess Parker singing "The Ballad of Davy Crockett."

I took the punishments pretty hard. I don't remember this, but one of my aunts later said she was visiting our house one time when Lou got angry at the boys. She shouted at us to get out of the house, to go play outside, to leave her in peace, and threw us all out the back door. The other boys went and played a game of some kind. But this aunt said that I went over by the fence and started crying, like I had my feelings hurt.

Could that be true? I guess so. I wanted Lou's affection. I wanted her to like me. I called her "Mom," because that seemed like the right thing to do. I wanted her to treat me like her son, the way she treated George, to love me and be proud of me and all that.

But that's not the way she was—at least not with me. She wasn't very affectionate. She didn't hug her boys, or kiss them, or tell them she loved them. In fact, I don't remember her being affectionate with my father, either. I never saw them being loving toward each other. That just wasn't their way.

My dad wasn't very physical, at least in a good way, either. I remember him holding me when I was a baby, because I remember his scratchy beard. I didn't like his beard. I liked being held by my mother, because she was soft and gentle. With my father, it was rough. I remember him pushing me on the swings when I was really little, and I remember it hurt—he shoved. By the time he married Lou and moved us into the house on Hawthorne, the only kind of physical touching I got was the spanking.

The other boys later said they were scared of Lou and her temper. George remembered Lou getting hysterical. She would start yelling and screaming, and my dad would have to grab her hands and hold them in order not to get hit. "She was a screamer," George said. "When she started yelling, you got to it. You set the table without being asked twice. You jumped."

Brian remembered the same thing. "There were serious amounts of yelling in our family, and terrible arguments," he said. "They drove me into my own little zone. My reaction was to just withdraw. I used to go to bed early on purpose, so I wouldn't be around it."

Unlike me, the other boys never seemed to do anything wrong, or never seemed to get in trouble for it. Brian was a good kid. He did what he was told, and stayed out of trouble. And George was smarter than me at avoiding detection. We'd do the same thing, but I'd get a spanking and he wouldn't. He was the favorite.

For example, Lou had strict rules about coming home from school. I had to come straight home or I'd get punished. But George could dawdle, hang out with friends, whatever. If I did that, I got sent to my room, or worse. I knew this wasn't fair, but I didn't know what to do about it. My dad wasn't home that much, and when he was home he didn't want to be bothered with a lot of stuff about "Lou hit me" or "Lou spanked me" or "It's not fair." When he came home, he might have time to give me a spanking, but not for a conversation about it.

So there wasn't any reason to go to him and complain about Lou. He didn't want to hear it.

I don't know when I started having trouble in school, but I did. I had the same trouble there that I had at home. I didn't like being told what to do. I didn't like *rules*. I liked doing what I liked doing, but I didn't like doing what I didn't like doing. I did well in the subjects that interested me, but that was it. I'd get bored, and I'd get into trouble. It wasn't malicious stuff. It was just stuff a kid does when he's bored or wants attention.

The school was typical of California schools of that time. It was a collection of one-story bungalows—stucco buildings painted an institutional beige—connected by walkways that were covered like a carport. Between each building was a planted area. Behind the school was a large grassy field.

I'd sit in those bungalows, staring out the window, thinking about things I'd rather be doing, wishing I could go outside and play. I was bored. I didn't feel challenged. So I got into trouble.

Like one time, in the third grade, I took a black crayon and colored in the area around my eye. I made up a story about what happened. When I went home I told Lou that I fell down on this crayon and it colored my eye in.

I got a big spanking for that one.

Another time we had a rainstorm. It started coming down in buckets. For some reason our teacher was out of the room. Suddenly I wanted to be out of the room, too. So I just left. I went outside and ran down to the athletic field and stood in the rain. I got soaked to the skin, and I got sent home.

I got a big spanking for that one, too.

Another time I was running down the walkway between the classrooms and I ran into a post and split my head open. I got in trouble for that, too—not for splitting my head open, but for running.

My behavior was a bigger problem, for me and the school, because my dad was a teacher at Hillview. Everybody knew whose kid I was. So when I did something bad it got noticed. It must have been embarrassing for my father to have his kid in trouble all the time. There were many after-school discussions about Howard in the teachers' lounge.

Like I said, I never did anything bad. I didn't get into fights. Later on, I would start stealing things for real, but then I was just high-spirited.

I wasn't a stupid kid, and I didn't get bad grades. I got A's and B's in history and art, because they interested me. I liked to draw. I liked to make things up. I liked stories, too. I was interested in the Old West. (I thought of myself as someone who would have lived in the Old West—that outlaw thing.) But if a subject didn't interest me, I didn't make any effort, so I got C's and D's.

I wish I had saved my report cards. Only one survives from that period. It's for seventh-grade math, from the first quarter of the school year in 1960. I was eleven. I got a B. What's surprising is that in the "Work Habits" and "Citizenship" categories I got mostly satisfactory or excellent marks. I was satisfactory in things like "workmanship," "self-control," "courtesy" and "obeys school rules." I was excellent in "reliability" and "promptness."

I shouldn't be surprised by the B. I was pretty fast with numbers, and I was very good at games that involved logic. I was a good card player, a good checkers player, and an excellent chess player. I could beat most people at checkers, and by the time I was six or seven I could beat anybody at chess. My brothers and my father stopped playing with me because they couldn't win.

Maybe if I had developed more of an interest in things like that—things that challenged my brain—I could have stayed out of trouble at school and at home. But I couldn't stay out of trouble. I was always doing something that made Lou mad. Sometimes, she got *real* mad. And then she got violent.

One time, when we lived on Hawthorne, Lou hurt me so bad that it scared my dad. He told me later that one afternoon when he was coming home from work, he knew there was trouble at home before he got out of the car. Halfway down the block he could hear this horrible screaming. He ran into the house to find me in the bedroom, pinned down by Lou, one arm twisted behind my back, yelling my head off.

Another time, Lou was cutting all the boys' hair. I was last. I was sitting on a little stool, waiting for her to finish. She was cleaning up, using an old Electrolux vacuum cleaner to pick up the hair. For some reason, she took the metal end of the vacuum cleaner hose and hit me on the top of my head with it.

I flinched.

She said, "Oh, did that hurt?"

I said no. I wouldn't admit that anything hurt.

So she hit me again, but harder this time. I flinched again. She said, "How about that? Did that hurt?"

I said no.

So she hit me again, real hard this time. I felt dizzy. She said, "How about *that*? Did *that* hurt?"

I didn't answer. I figured if I said no again she'd hit me again. I thought she was going to knock me out.

The last time she ever really spanked me was about a year after that.

She had gotten mad at me about something—it could have been anything—and she made me go to my room. Then she came up there to give me a spanking. She usually had something with her when she did this, like a paddle or a wooden spoon. Her hands were too small to do any damage. It used to scare me to see her come into the room carrying a wooden spoon, because I knew what she was going to do with it.

But this time, for some reason, I didn't care. I wasn't afraid. She looked small to me. She looked weak. So when she started spanking me, I started laughing. It didn't hurt. It wasn't scary. It was funny.

When she stopped, I didn't say anything to her. I stopped laughing, and I glared. I stood up to her for the first time. After that, I was punished only by my dad. Lou knew I wouldn't laugh when *he* spanked me.

I was getting to be a big kid—too big for Lou to spank, too big for her to scare—and I think that must have scared *her*. It must have made her wonder, *What if he ever turns on me?* I never raised my hand to her, and hardly ever raised my voice, but she must have wondered what would happen if I ever fought back. Because I was big, and because she hated me, that must have been a frightening thought.

She'd have to find another way to keep me in line.

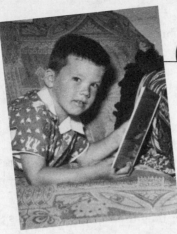

Chapter 3

762 Edgewood

In the summer of 1957, when I was nine years old, we moved house again. I don't know where they got the money, or how they afforded it, but my father and Lou traded in the two-bedroom Hawthorne bungalow for a huge, seven-bedroom mansion, a one-hundred-year-old Queen Anne Victorian, at 762 Edgewood. It was only a couple of miles away from the house on Hawthorne, but it was as different as night and day. My father later remembered that he and Lou sold the Hawthorne house for about $12,000, and bought the Edgewood house for about $25,000—a lot of money for a guy who was making only $4,000 a year, with a wife who didn't work.

The house had an interesting history. It had been built in 1840, when there was nothing but oak trees for hundreds of yards in every direction, and was owned by a member of the Winchester family. These Winchesters had built their fortune on the famous rifle made by the Winchester Repeating Arms Company—the gun that won the West.

The Winchester house on Edgewood was miles away from that other Winchester house—the Winchester Mystery House, which had a strange history. It was owned by the widow of the original gun company owner, and she was construction-crazy. She started building the house in the 1880s, and kept workers going around the clock for more than forty years. The house, which turned into a big tourist attraction, was seven stories tall and was supposed to be haunted.

The Winchester house on Edgewood wasn't haunted until *we* moved into it. It was just a big old house. It was two stories, not seven. The paint was peeling. Some of the woodwork was sagging. Some of the shingles were missing.

But to me the house was beautiful. It sat on an enormous piece of property and was hidden from the street by big pepper trees, oak trees, pine trees, and fig trees that were great for climbing and building tree houses and forts. It had a big front porch, a sun porch, and a sewing porch. There were oak floors and a huge oak front door, and a mahogany banister going up to the second floor. (You could really get in trouble if you got caught sliding down that banister.) There were six bedrooms upstairs—I had my own bedroom, next to Brian's—and two bathrooms. There were five fireplaces, too. We always had a fire going in the living room and the dining room—partly because my dad liked fires, and partly to save on heating bills. I spent a lot of time out in the backyard chopping wood for those fireplaces.

There was a big bay window in the living room that looked out onto the front yard, and tall windows on the second floor, and two round port-hole windows on the side of the house near the garage. There was a spooky attic above that.

I slept upstairs, on the side of the house closest to the garage. For the first time since I was a little boy at Spartan Village, when I was still an only child, I had my own room. I had my own closet. I had some privacy.

But it was also creepy. Going to bed by myself was kind of scary. The house *felt* haunted. At night when it was windy or raining, the house felt like a ship rolling on the sea. The tree branches would scrape against the side of the house. On Hawthorne I had been bothered by fears of what was around me when I slept. I thought the floor was crawling with alligators, or snakes, or spiders, and they were coming to bite me. Now I'd lie awake at night and hear these noises and be sure something was coming to get me—monsters, vampires, kidnappers, you name it. Like I said before, I was a kid with a vivid imagination, and at night my imagination turned against me. My mind did a lot of scary things with that old house.

Television didn't help. There were always creepy movies on TV, starring Boris Karloff or Bela Lugosi. Things like that got inside my head and gave me terrible nightmares.

Other than being afraid, living in the new house was pretty good. The yard had all kinds of places to play. George and I made up games, and had lots of room for cowboys and Indians, or army. We spent a lot of time climbing those trees. Binky, who was into cars and had a hot rod that he liked to work on, dug a pit in the backyard, a kind of work bay like they have in gas stations where you can go under the car without having to lie down on your back. He'd do his lube jobs and oil changes and stuff down there. George and I used that as a fort when Binky wasn't around.

The backyard was a home for our dog, Monster, a short-haired mutt that moved with us from Hawthorne. It was also a place for discipline. My dad had all kinds of plans for landscaping and gardening there, and we were his work crew. If we'd done something wrong, he'd sentence us to picking weeds. He'd take two stakes and drive them into the ground and stretch a string between them. He'd say, "I want you boys to clear out all the weeds from here to that string."

It didn't take me and George long to figure out the solution to *that* problem. You'd just wait until Dad wasn't looking, then pull up the stakes and put them back into the ground closer to the house. You'd be done in no time! My dad always seemed surprised that we got finished so soon.

I was in the fifth grade when we moved to Edgewood. Soon after that, our family situation started changing. First Binky moved out. He went to live with his dad and his dad's new wife. Around the same time, we found out Lou was pregnant. A short time later, she gave birth to a boy she and my father named Kirk, after a doctor of their acquaintance. He was a sweet-tempered little blond kid.

Now we were a proper Los Altos family, so we had to keep up appearances.

On Hawthorne, things had been a little loose. There was that homemade third bedroom, where Binky slept. There was that homemade swimming pool. When my dad decided to build that, he tore down the old split-rail fence and put the swimming pool right in the front yard. He hung a sign on it that said, WE DON'T SWIM IN YOUR TOILET, SO PLEASE DON'T PEE IN OUR POOL.

But now we were Los Altos people, living in a real Los Altos house. It had been owned by the *Winchesters*. There wasn't going to be any pool in the front yard on Edgewood. We were hardly allowed to even *play* in the front yard. In fact, by order of Lou, we were not allowed to go out the front door at all. When we wanted to go outside to the front of the house, we had to use the service entrance.

Moving to Edgewood meant we had to dress differently, too. That was part of keeping up appearances. We lived among the rich people now. So Lou and my dad made me wear corduroy pants and a button-down shirt to school every day. Green corduroy pants and a green corduroy jacket! I was nine years old. What happened to blue jeans and a T-shirt? That's what all the other kids were wearing. That's what I wanted to wear. That's what every kid in America wanted to wear. We wanted to look like James Dean, not Little Lord Fauntleroy.

But we were keeping up appearances.

Lou began to furnish the house nicely, too. She had a thing for cherrywood furniture, and she'd search antique stores and estate sales and barn sales looking for affordable pieces. Soon the downstairs part of our mansion really looked like a mansion. Needless to say, we were told to keep off the cherrywood furniture, never to touch the cherrywood furniture.

Lou was really obsessive about things like that. She had all kinds of rules about keeping the house clean. You could not go into the dining room at all. The furniture was special and expensive and you weren't allowed to touch it. You could walk from the living room to the kitchen, or vice versa, but never through the dining room. We were also supposed to stay out of each other's rooms, and we were never allowed into her sewing room.

The dinner table rules became stricter, too. You weren't allowed to speak at the dinner table unless you were spoken to. You were supposed to keep your elbows off the table and your napkin in your lap. Mealtimes were tense.

If my dad was home for dinner, he'd demand a full report of your day: What happened at school? Did you do your homework? Otherwise, we ate dinner almost without speaking. Lou would dish it out and we'd sit, me and George and Brian and Lou, without talking. If we did something wrong, we'd get punished.

For me, moving to Edgewood, everything changed and nothing changed. I was still the same person. So, I did things wrong and I got punished. I spent a lot of time in my room. Lou didn't like my table manners. She didn't like how rambunctious I was—and being in the big fancy house on Edgewood, the Winchester house, with all that cherrywood furniture, made it worse. I think I was embarrassing to her. Like, a lady with a beautiful Victorian house on Edgewood should have children with beautiful manners.

I didn't have beautiful manners. No one had ever taught me beautiful manners. I was a big kid, and I was a hungry kid, and when it was time to eat I got busy. I chowed down.

Lou didn't like that. She didn't like me goofing off with George, or picking on Brian, or making jokes at the dinner table.

So she started making me eat dinner alone. I'd eat in the breakfast nook, before the other kids ate. I'd be sent to my room while the rest of the kids had their dinner. Some nights we weren't together at all. I'd get my supper in the kitchen. Then Lou would serve something to Brian and George. She'd feed the baby upstairs. Then my dad would come home late and eat in the living room, in front of the TV. By then I would usually have been sent to my room for something or other.

I remember feeling very sad a lot of the time, and left out. I could hear the TV going downstairs. I could hear Brian and George laughing, watching *Disneyland* or *Father Knows Best*. I could hear the theme music from *Gunsmoke* or *Peter Gunn* or *Dragnet*. I felt isolated, and lonely, and unhappy. And *mad*. It wasn't fair.

I was always being punished for doing things that my brothers did. I didn't get rewarded the way my brothers did, either—especially George. When my dad built the swimming pool on Hawthorne, George got swimming lessons. I had to learn on my own. When we moved to Edgewood, George got a new ten-speed bike. I got a bike that my father had bought used and then re-painted himself.

What was so special about George? What was so bad about me? How come I didn't deserve a new bike?

Years later I found out that George's special stuff came from his dad—Red Cox. George spent a lot of weekends visiting with Red and his new wife, and for Christmas or his birthday he'd get things like that new bike, or a new baseball glove—from his dad. His dad had paid for his swimming lessons. If someone had explained that to me, I might have understood. But no one told me.

So naturally enough I imagined that I got treated like a second-class citizen because I *was* a second-class citizen. I thought they just didn't love me as much as they loved George. I wasn't good enough.

This wasn't the whole story, of course. I found out years later that Red never paid much child support or alimony. The gifts he gave George might have been flashy, but there weren't very many of them. George told me later that his dad wasn't into Christmas, or birthdays, and sometimes didn't get him anything at all. He also told me that his father was a real alcoholic, who would sometimes get drunk and stay drunk for days at a time. (Alcoholism ran all over that family. Red's father was a drunk, too, George said. So was Lou's father. George said he figured out in his early twenties that he'd better be careful with alcohol himself, or he'd wind up an alcoholic, too.)

I was jealous of George going off with his dad on the weekends.

I shouldn't have been. Sometimes he was afraid to even get in the car with Red. "I remember begging him not to take me anywhere," George said. "He'd come over and he'd give me a hug and I could smell how much he'd been drinking. I'd say, 'Please don't get in the car.' I was scared."

If I had known any of that, I might have felt different. I might have understood that George's life wasn't as perfect as it looked.

But that would have left me with Brian to compare myself to, and that wouldn't have worked out, either. For his eighth birthday, he got pony rides. My parents hired someone to come to the house with a pony for the little boys and a real horse for the bigger boys. I was so excited, because I was a big cowboy kind of guy and I thought horses were great. But Lou wouldn't even let me go and see them. She said, "It's Brian's birthday, not yours, and you're not invited." I couldn't even go and touch the horses. I had to stay upstairs, in my room, while Brian and his friends took rides around the backyard.

Maybe that's part of why I behaved badly. I was being treated like a bad boy, so I acted like a bad boy. The rules weren't fair, so I broke the rules.

The weird thing is, I don't remember anyone ever sitting down and asking me what was going on. I got yelled at. I got called names. Lou called me "moron" or "idiot." My dad would say, "Don't be stupid," or, "Stop acting like a jerk." I got threatened. I got punished. But no one ever *talked* to me. No one ever asked me what was going on.

No one at school did, either. Maybe they didn't have time. In those days, the population in our area was growing so fast that the schools couldn't handle it. It was the beginning of the baby boom, and there wasn't room for all the boomers. Hillview, like a lot of other elementary schools, was on a split schedule. Half the kids would start in the early morning and come home in the early afternoon. The other half would start in the late morning and come home in the late afternoon. There were six first-grade classes at Hillview at one time—three in the morning, three in the afternoon. So, even though my stepbrother George was only three months older than me, we were never in the same class together. I'd have to get up early and get out to the street to catch the school bus for the early session. He could get up later, and he got to walk to school. How come he got to walk to school, and walk home? I don't know. But *I* had to take that dumb bus.

Just like at home, I think, the teachers and administrators were so overwhelmed that they never had time to single me out except for punishment. Nowadays there would be a school psychologist who specialized in kids like me. I'd probably be diagnosed as hyperactive, or having attention deficit disorder. In those days, it was just easier to punish me.

At home, no one ever played with me, either. In the evenings we'd watch TV shows like *The Danny Thomas Show* or *The Donna Reed Show*. I'd see those families and wonder what was wrong with ours, or what was wrong with me. My dad didn't teach me how to ride a bike, or throw a ball. I don't ever remember doing any of that stuff with him. He didn't sit down for heart-to-heart talks with me. He was either away, at work, or he was at home and tired. In most of my memories of him from that time he was either mad at me, ignoring me, or sending me out to the backyard to chop wood.

Most of the time he sent me out there alone. But not always. Almost the only times I remember us spending time together were when we were working. Even though I was only nine or ten, I was big, and I was strong. So he'd make me do certain work projects with him that the other boys couldn't do.

One year he decided to pave our long, curvy driveway with fresh asphalt. He rented a trailer and picked up a load of asphalt. When he got home, we'd shovel it out, smooth it out, and tamp it down. Then he'd go get another load. We spent a whole weekend paving the driveway out to the street.

Another time he decided to replace the sewer line from the house to the street. I spent forever out there with a shovel, digging the trench for the new sewer line, all the way from the house, across the yard, to the street. It was hard work, and I probably wasn't big enough and strong enough to be doing it. I got blisters. I made mistakes. He yelled at me. I hated it. It wasn't like some bonding experience where we worked together and talked about life and love and sports and politics. It wasn't like that at all. It was hard, hot, sweaty work that we did without talking to each other.

Another time I remember we were cutting wood together. He was using a sledgehammer and a metal wedge to split a log. Suddenly a big chunk of the metal wedge broke off and hit me in the shoulder. I felt like I'd been shot by a bullet, and I looked like I'd been stabbed. It hurt a lot and it bled a lot. But I remember him saying, "Stop crying, you baby. It's nothing."

I wasn't the only one he scared. My cousin Linda Pickering told me later that when she was young, her mother was mentally unstable. She was in and out of mental institutions. The kids—Linda was the oldest of six children—would be alone in the house. Sometimes my dad would come over on a weekend morning to take charge. He would start shouting at them, telling them it was wrong for them to sleep late on a Saturday, and yelling at them to get out of bed and do their chores. Linda said this happened more than once. She was sure her mother hadn't asked Rod to do this. Maybe it was the only way he knew to try to be helpful to his struggling sister-in-law.

My dad was working hard, two or three jobs at a time, but it was still hard for him to support his family. One time he and Lou got behind on their payments on the Hawthorne house, and almost had it taken away from them. There was more than one letter to a creditor asking for patience, asking for relief, promising to keep up with the payments. In one I've seen, my dad says he is "financially embarrassed," and writes in his steady schoolteacher hand, "If you will permit me to make smaller payments for the next month or two I will be able to make my tax payment on time and not further complicate my financial situation. I am enclosing a check for twenty-five dollars . . ."

That must have been hard for my dad. He grew up in the Depression, without a father, moving from town to town, being pushed off onto his relatives, while his mother tried to make enough to raise her sons. He had always been careful about money. He never drove a new car. He never bought fancy clothes. So that's how we lived, too. We hardly ever ate out in restaurants. Nothing was ever bought new if it could be bought used, and nothing was ever paid for if it could be had for free. Even the lumber he used for his building projects was wood that he scavenged off the streets, out of trash bins or off construction sites.

Having my dad work a lot was bad for me. When he was gone, I was left alone with Lou. One time, when we were still living on Hawthorne, he went to Fort Sill, Oklahoma, for some National Guard training. I know it was November, because he was gone for my birthday. I remember having a birthday party. It was my eighth birthday. I had some friends from the neighborhood come over for cake and ice cream, with Hershey's chocolate sauce.

I had also invited a little girl from the neighborhood. I liked her. But I was nervous to have her come to the party. George and some of the other boys had found out that she'd show you her underpants if you gave her a cookie. So George was always giving her cookies and fooling around with her. He tried to get me to do it, too, but I was too embarrassed. I wouldn't play along.

I wanted her to come to the party, but I was afraid George and the other boys from the neighborhood would say bad things about her, or make fun of her.

I was also scared because Lou was in charge. But it seemed to go pretty well. Then after the cake and ice cream the boys started picking on the little girl. I was afraid they were going to start picking on me, too. So I got out of the way. I didn't stick up for her. No one did. It ended up being an unhappy birthday for me.

My dad was gone for almost a month. Without him there, Lou was on top of me for everything. I couldn't catch a break. It seemed like I spent the whole time getting yelled at and sent to my room and spanked or hit or punished. Lou would yell at me to get out of the kitchen, get out of the house, get out of her way, or stop doing this or that. Then, if I didn't move quickly enough, or if I gave her any guff, I'd get punished. Half the time I didn't even know what I was being punished for. I was just *bad*.

And all that punishing still didn't satisfy her. When my dad got back from Fort Sill, she told him that she couldn't handle me anymore, that he had to do something with me. So, to keep the peace in the family, my dad started sending me to spend the weekends with his uncle Orville and aunt Evelyn.

I didn't know it at the time, but they weren't really his uncle and aunt. They weren't family at all. Evelyn was the former housekeeper who my dad and my uncle Kenny had lived with in that logging camp when they were in high school. Her husband, Orville, had been a lumber man. He had worked for Long Bell Logging, in Ryderwood, Washington.

By now, Orville and Evelyn were living in Mountain View, another suburb of San Jose, where they had a little one-bedroom apartment on Camille Court. Evelyn had a job on a ranch, sorting eggs. Orville was the custodian at Springer Elementary School in Mountain View, where he was very well liked by all the kids. I'd go over there on Saturday and spend the weekend helping him at Springer, and helping my aunt with Sunday school. They were nice people, and they were very nice to me.

My uncle Kenny said that Orville and Evelyn weren't able to have children. But they loved kids, so they loved having me around. Orville, like my dad, had lost a parent early in life. His mother had died giving birth to him, and his father sort of disappeared. And so, like Lou, he was raised mostly by his grandparents.

I liked Orville and Evelyn a lot. They didn't criticize me all the time. Orville and I could talk about men stuff—sports and camping and fishing—and he never talked down to me. He and Evelyn asked me to help out, and I helped out, and that made me feel useful and appreciated.

They belonged to the St. Paul Lutheran Church, and they were serious about religion, which was a new thing for me. My family went to church on Easter, and my grandmother had some ideas she got from Christian Science, but that was it. Religion didn't enter our house at all. My dad used to make fun of it. He'd say, "The Bible—what's the big deal? I could've written that."

Orville would say, "Too bad, Rod—you're missing out on a lot of royalties."

I don't know whose idea it was, but someone taught me how to pray and got me doing it when I was real young. There's a picture of me dated July 1956. I'm lying on my back in a wood-paneled room, with my hands folded together, and I'm praying. There's a crucifix on the wall. It looks like I'm in a cabin, which might mean I was on vacation up in the mountains. If the date on the picture is right, I was seven and a half years old.

When we weren't doing church stuff, Orville and Evelyn took me to do things that were fun. We went to the rodeo over at Steven's Creek, and we went miniature golfing. We went out to dinner and had hamburgers or pizza.

With my dad, we hardly went out for dinner at all, and we didn't go to fun places too often. I remember once going to a place that served steak. I was pretty interested in that steak. Maybe my brothers were, too. But my dad said, "No, you wouldn't like that. You're getting hamburgers." Then *he* had the steak.

He was strict about things like that. Sometimes we'd go down to Clint's, the ice cream place, for an ice cream cone. But you couldn't just get whatever flavor you wanted. It had to be vanilla, chocolate, or strawberry. You couldn't order another flavor. My dad wouldn't let you. I wanted to try licorice ice cream. That sounded great! But he said no. Ice cream wasn't *supposed* to taste like licorice. It wasn't right, and he wasn't buying it.

Every once in a while we'd go to a park, or to the beach— someplace free, because it had to be someplace free. There was a park over near Santa Cruz that we went to a lot. It had a rock you could slide down into the water.

The only big trip I remember us taking was a really big one. In 1955, the summer that it opened, we went to Disneyland.

I don't remember many details about it, but my stepbrother George says we borrowed my uncle Kenny's new Buick—Dad's car wasn't dependable enough for the long, hot drive—and hit the road. We stayed at the Figueroa Hotel in downtown Los Angeles because the hotels around Disneyland were too expensive. When we got to the park, we found out that we weren't allowed to go on some of the rides because we were too small. Binky went on things like the Autopia ride, but me and George were too little for that. George mostly remembers going on the Rocket to the Moon ride. Bink convinced him during the takeoff that we really *were* going to the moon, and that we weren't coming back. George got scared and started crying. I think we were both seven years old.

What I remember most is that we weren't allowed to do a lot of the things we wanted to do. Some rides cost extra, so those were out—like the pirate-ship ride. We got our pictures taken on the dock, next to the pirate ship, but that was as close as we got. I remember having to stomp my feet to get on the rocket ride, too. At first my dad wasn't going to let me go on it, probably because it cost extra.

In the snapshots I've seen of that day we all look unhappy—like we don't want to stand around taking pictures, but we do want to get back on the rides—except my dad. He looks cheerful in every family photo I've ever seen. He's smiling like he's taken one of his famous "what-the-hell" pills. He used to joke about that. When something difficult was going to take place, he'd say, "I better take my what-the-hell pills."

The only family vacation we took regularly was the one to Uncle Ross's cabin in the mountains. Even after my dad married Lou, we were still welcome there. Each spring, Uncle Ross would mail us the key to the front door, and we'd drive up there the weekend before Easter. We'd usually stay a whole week in that giant cabin.

It was a paradise for kids. The walls were hung with moose heads, elk heads, and deer antlers. The snow outside was always deep enough for skiing, and sometimes so deep that we'd have to shovel our way in, just to get to the front door.

I remember playing in the snow for hours with George. We'd put on ski boots and strap them into the skis—that's how long ago this was, before there were modern bindings—and ski for so long that we always wound up with blisters. When we were older, we'd sneak cigarettes and smoke them in the snow. We'd build snow forts.

George remembers this as the happiest time in our family. It probably wasn't too much of a treat for Lou. The house had a wood-burning fireplace for heat and a wood-burning stove for cooking. Her job was probably twice as hard as it was at home. But for us kids, it was a great place to be.

At home, sometimes my dad would take me for an outing, but we wouldn't go anywhere fun at all. He was just taking me out of the house to give Lou a break. Some evenings, for example, he'd take me with him to the National Guard Armory, on Hedding Street in San Jose. It was a big building with a wooden-floored gymnasium on the first floor and offices and meeting rooms on the second floor. He'd go up to the second floor to take care of his National Guard business, and leave me on my own down in the gym. Outside, it was a schoolboy's dream—a gigantic parking lot full of army trucks and jeeps. But inside it was just a gym with a polished-wood floor. No balls. No games. No one to play games with. It wasn't much fun for a kid. So, after a while I'd get whiny and start asking him to take me home. I'm sure he didn't like that.

As I got older, things at home got worse.

It was probably my fault, because I was jealous of the good treatment he got, but I stopped getting along with George. It seemed like he and I were opposites now. He liked the Los Angeles

Dodgers, and I liked the San Francisco Giants. He liked Elvis Presley, and I liked Ricky Nelson. He liked *Father Knows Best,* and I liked *Bachelor Father.* We didn't play together that much anymore, and when we did, we argued.

One time at school, I said something he didn't like and he jumped on me. We fell on the ground, wrestling like a couple of wildcats.

Lou had a weird way of dealing with fights. Instead of letting us work it out, she'd make us put on boxing gloves and go into the front yard. She'd referee the fight, and we'd go a few rounds until one of us had enough.

We did this more than once. It was stupid. I was much taller than George. I had a longer reach and I weighed more. Not that he wasn't tough—he was plenty tough. He was strong, and he was stocky. But I had the reach. All I had to do was keep him away from me until I got a clear shot.

I was pretty good at fighting, but I didn't like to fight. Some kids did. I knew guys who *looked* for fights. I wasn't one of those guys. I didn't like getting hurt, and I didn't like hurting other people.

Once, when I was about ten, I was with some of my cousins and some of their friends at my uncle Gene's house. We were in the yard, and we were wrestling, just like they did on TV. I picked up this kid and threw him—just like they did on TV. He got hurt, and I got in trouble. He went into the house crying. I was banned from wrestling.

Even now, it scares me. I could have hurt that kid bad. I could have broken his neck. It was a dangerous thing to do, and I sort of knew that at the time. But I didn't care. I didn't stop. I picked him up and threw him on the ground.

I still feel bad about that today. I could have been friends with that kid. Instead, I hurt him, and scared him, and got excluded from the rest of the games that day.

I got in trouble for that. I also got in trouble for lots of things I didn't do, sometimes for things George did. One time, Lou was cleaning up Kirk's baby toys. Some of them were wet, like someone had spit on them. She accused me of doing it, even though I told her I didn't, and gave me a spanking and sent me to my room. Later that day George came home and she told him what had happened. He confessed: He had spit on the toys himself. By then, Lou wasn't angry anymore. She had taken it out on me already. So she didn't punish George at all, and she didn't apologize to me.

I had suspected for a long time that I was getting the short end of the stick. When anything went wrong, I got blamed—and punished. But when George got caught red-handed, nothing happened. Now here was the proof. I wasn't crazy. I wasn't making things up. It was *true*. I couldn't catch a break.

Sometimes, when I thought I did something good, it turned out I had done something bad.

For example, George and I were on Little League baseball teams. We were both obsessed with baseball. I idolized guys like Juan Marichal, Warren Spahn, and Willie Mays. George later told me I was the better athlete of the two of us, even though he was more popular and usually got picked to play before I did when we were choosing up sides.

One time, my team played against George's team. It was a good game, and my team won. But I wasn't congratulated for playing well and winning the game. Instead, I was criticized for not cheering loud enough for George when he was up at bat. What kind of sportsmanship is that? Even if it is your brother, you don't cheer for the other team during the game.

I don't have only my own memory to rely on when it comes to my childhood. George would tell me, much later in my life, that it was just as bad as I remembered it.

He remembers Lou telling me, in front of the family, in front of my dad, things like, "You make me sick. You eat like a pig. Let me go get you a trough." She'd say, "You eat like an animal. I'm going to get you a shovel."

If I asked for a second helping of something, she'd get mad at me. George remembers me complaining about going to bed hungry—and getting caught if I did something about it. There was a big cookie jar in the kitchen, with a heavy screw-top lid on it. George would go and get a cookie if he wanted one, and nobody said a word. But if I went into the kitchen and Lou heard that screw-top lid being opened, she'd come screaming in there and tell me to leave the cookies alone.

I don't remember Lou ever doing anything that seemed like fun. She didn't enjoy herself much. She did have an accordion, though, a great big old-fashioned one that she kept locked in a box. Every once in a while she'd take it out and sit by herself, playing accordion music. I thought she played very well, and I liked listening to her. But she almost never played. She almost never had any fun.

Mostly, it seemed like, she worried and got angry. My cousin Linda remembers going to the beach at Santa Cruz with Lou and her sons. They'd spread a blanket on the sand. Linda would run down to the water. But as soon as Cleon or George would leave the blanket, Lou would start yelling at them to be careful, to not go near the water, to not get dirty.

George remembers her being neurotic about cleanliness, too, and also remembers her inspecting my underwear. If she found anything in there, any stains, I got a beating. George remembers Lou screaming her head off, dragging me up the stairs by one arm on the way to giving me a beating.

I got lots of beatings.

"Mom would start and Pop would finish it when he came home," George said. "You had bruises on your body almost every day of your life. You had marks all over you."

George felt guilty about it. Brian did, too. He said, "I was no threat to anyone, and no competition for anyone, and I was adored. No one had to punish me." He and George never got hit. Especially George. My dad was not allowed to touch him, criticize him, or punish him in any way. Brian never did anything bad, and Lou refused to punish George, no matter what he got caught doing. So he felt bad when he saw me getting a beating for something he was probably doing himself.

"I knew they were hurting you and I knew it was wrong," he told me later. "And I know that if it happened today, someone would be going to jail."

Was it all bad? It couldn't have been. Sometimes I wonder if I just remember the bad things. Brian says he doesn't ever remember happy times, living in that house with me and George and Lou and Dad. Could we all have forgotten some of the stuff that was good?

My stepbrother George remembers some of the good things. He remembers Lou helping us build a tree fort. He remembers her buying us paint-by-numbers kits, and taking us to the library.

I don't remember that. I don't even remember celebrating most of my birthdays. George remembers one year I got three of the same gift, a board game called Calling All Cars. We kept one and took back two. Birthdays weren't anything special. You'd get a gift, but it was usually clothes or a book. That was the one thing that my father and Lou weren't cheap about. There were always books around. They would buy books, new books. You could always get a book. Lou would bake a cake. I didn't like her cakes much, but it was nice to get a cake just the same.

Christmas wasn't a big deal, either. There weren't a bunch of presents. We didn't have a giant Christmas tree with a mountain of gifts under it. It was almost like a regular day, except that you'd get a baseball mitt (used, always) or something like that.

I do remember that I was the only kid in the family who got new clothes that were really new. Everyone else got hand-me-downs. There was no one big enough whose hand-me-downs I could wear. So I usually got new clothes and new shoes.

I don't remember hearing anything during that period about my little brother Bruce. He had survived and was adopted by my father's uncle Frank and his wife Bea, who lived up in Centralia, Washington. But I do remember seeing him one time. He was at one of my uncles' house—either Kenneth's or Gene's. He must have been seven or eight years old by then. He would stand and put his left foot in front of his right foot and rock back and forth and make a little noise. He couldn't talk. He couldn't recognize his own name. He could walk if you helped him. Otherwise, he would just stand and rock back and forth. He didn't seem unhappy, or happy, or anything. He was just sort of there.

Seeing him made me sad. It reminded me about my mother. It must have reminded my dad about her, too. Brian believed this was why Bruce never lived with us—because my father couldn't bear to be reminded about the death of his wife. He later told me that he never saw Bruce again after that day at my uncle's house.

With all of this trouble at home, it's no surprise that I was starting to get into trouble away from home, too.

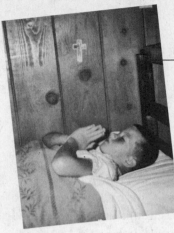

Chapter 4

Trouble

There was a five-and-dime store in Los Altos called Sprouse Ritz—part of the chain of variety stores, like Woolworth, that were all over the country. The store was right in downtown Los Altos, and it had a front door and a back door. If you were smart about it, you could go in one door, pocket something quick, and go out the other door and not get caught. I got to be pretty good at stealing things.

But I also got caught stealing things. One of the first times, I got caught by my own father. He saw me playing with a yo-yo. It was a beautiful yo-yo, the classic yellow Duncan Butterfly. My dad knew he hadn't bought me the yo-yo. He probably knew I didn't have enough money to buy it myself. He asked me to show it to him.

"That's some yo-yo," he said. "Where'd you get it?"

"I bought it, down at Sprouse Ritz."

"How much was it?"

I wasn't stupid. I knew how much a yo-yo cost. He couldn't catch me like that. So I told him, "One ninety-nine."

"And tax?" he asked. "How much was the tax?"

Well, he had me there. I knew how much a yo-yo was, but I didn't know how much the sales tax was. He knew I'd stolen it. He took it away from me.

First he punished me. I got spanked. Then he told me I was

grounded. I wasn't going to be allowed to go out and play for maybe a week. Then he told me we were going back to Sprouse Ritz to return the yo-yo.

I think he called the store in advance, because they didn't seem that surprised to see me or hear why I was there. We went into the store and marched up to the counter, and I handed over the yo-yo and explained I had stolen it. My father stood somewhere in the back of the store—near enough that he would have known if I'd just dropped the yo-yo on the counter and taken off.

That was pretty humiliating, but it wasn't my only yo-yo shoplifting incident. Another time I was in this little store where I was stealing candy. I had my pockets stuffed with candy. I started to leave but the lady behind the counter caught me.

"Come here," she said. "Empty your pockets."

I was busted. I took all the stuff out of my pockets—candy, chocolate, bubble gum—and put it on the counter.

"And the yo-yo," the lady said.

Then she looked at the yo-yo. It wasn't new. It wasn't in the package. It belonged to me. She thought I had stolen it, but now she saw she was wrong.

"All right," she said. "Never mind. Get your stuff and get out of here."

So I filled my pockets back up with all that candy and took my yo-yo and left.

Usually I did my criminal things with a partner. I wasn't a brave thief. I had to have a partner in crime, someone working with me on the big jobs. That's what I did with the great train robbery.

It was actually a train *station* robbery. The train used to run along what's now Foothill Expressway. The Los Altos depot is still there, right down the street from Whitecliff Market, where my dad worked after school.

There were some newspaper racks at that little train station. We'd have to cross the tracks to get from our house to the elementary school or the junior high, or to go to town. So we went by the station all the time. That's how I got the idea of robbing the news-paper racks.

Me and a friend of mine named Danny figured out that, even though there were sometimes people around there, usually no one was watching the newspaper racks. So I'd be lookout. I'd stroll around the station, keeping an eye out for the cops, while Danny went and turned the newspaper racks upside down and spilled out all the coins. Then he'd turn the racks right side up, collect the coins, and we'd get out of there. We'd take the coins and turn them into toys and candy. We never made a lot of money, but it was enough for two ten-year-olds to keep themselves stuffed with chocolate and candy bars.

After we'd been doing this for a while and not getting caught, I got lazy. One day I decided no one was looking—without check-ing to see if no one was looking. Three cops jumped out and grabbed me and Danny. That landed us in the Los Altos police sta-tion. We were questioned, then my dad came to pick me up and take me home.

For some reason, instead of pressing charges, the cops and the newspaper people and my dad made a deal. I would get a paper route, and I would deliver the *San Francisco Examiner* until I'd paid all the money back.

Now I had a job. I got some of those newspaper bags to hang on my bicycle handlebars, and every morning before school I had a paper route.

I didn't like to work. And I didn't like getting up in the morn-ing. But the paper route was okay. It gave me a chance to do some-thing on my own, with no one looking over my shoulder. I got to go off by myself. I liked being by myself. With other people around, it was easy to get into trouble. When I was off on my own, I never had any problems. I never got into trouble. Well, usually I didn't, except when I was bored.

• • •

My dad started taking me to work with him at night, probably to get me out of the house and out of Lou's way. He'd drive me into Palo Alto to the Eastman Kodak processing plant. There was a big employees' parking lot. He'd park the car and tell me to stay in it until he got back.

I think he worked a six-hour shift. That was a long time to leave a ten-year-old kid in a car by himself and expect him to behave. I'd be okay for a while—doing my homework, or reading, or whatever—but then I'd get bored. I'd get out of the car and cruise around the parking lot and stare into the parked cars. I saw lots of interesting things in those cars. So, one night, I took some. I found a cool cigarette lighter. I found a yo-yo, and some sunglasses. I found a very nice eight-ball gear-shift knob that screwed on and off. I filled my pockets with this stuff, and then took it all back to my dad's car to play with.

I realized that my dad would notice if I had a pocket full of stolen items. So before he came back I hid them all under the seat, where he wouldn't see them. I figured I'd sneak them out of the car another time, when we were back home and he wasn't looking.

My dad finished his shift and came out to the car, and we drove home. As soon as he hit the brakes, stuff started rolling out from under the seat. He said, "What's that?" It didn't take him long to figure out what had happened. My dad had to return the stuff to the cars I'd stolen it from.

At school, too, I was in trouble a lot of the time. I was a cutup. I was bored. The more routine school stuff didn't interest me. When we had multiple-choice tests where you're supposed to fill in the boxes, I'd just fill in the boxes so they made an interesting pattern. *There. That looks nice!*

I didn't want to be a good student. I didn't want people to think I was a nerd. My dad was a teacher at the school. I didn't want to be perceived as Mr. Dully's little goody-goody son. So I was wild.

By the fall of 1960, I'd graduated from Hillview and moved to Covington, the local junior high school.

It was almost as close to our house as Hillview. I could walk there. I didn't have to ride the bus. Even better, on the way to school there were lots of fruit trees, especially apricots. I could eat my fill of 'cots before I even got to school. That made it easier not to steal other kids' lunches. I wasn't arriving at school hungry every day.

Junior high was a little scary. Covington was the big time. They had initiation at Covington, and every kid in Los Altos knew about it before he got there. If you were a new kid coming into the seventh grade, you knew it could happen to you. They would take a guy and strip him, and run his underwear up the flagpole. You did *not* want to be that kid. Or they'd hold you down and put butch wax in your hair and brush it straight up, and they'd roll your pant legs up above your calves. You had to stay that way all day long or you'd get beat up.

I was afraid that was going to happen to me. But it didn't—I think because I was so big that everyone thought I was an eighth- or ninth-grader who had transferred from another school. Initiation was just for seventh-graders. I got off easy.

I looked big for my age, and I was trying to seem older than I was, too. I had already started smoking.

It was George who first got me started on it. He would steal cigarettes from Lou. She had a cute artsy-craftsy box on the kitchen wall that held her cigarettes and her matches. George would steal them and take them into the backyard. We'd go around the back of the garage, or we'd go hide in The Pit—that hole in the backyard that Binky had dug to work on his car and that we had converted to a fort.

But he made fun of the way I smoked. I didn't inhale. I couldn't inhale. I wanted to, but I couldn't figure out how, even though he tried to teach me. He showed me how to French inhale, and how to blow smoke rings, but I couldn't get it. So he'd tease me and laugh at me.

We were bold about stealing the cigarettes. Lou was absent-minded, and sometimes she'd light a cigarette in the kitchen, set it in an ashtray, and then leave the room without it. We'd grab it and smoke it right there—snatch a couple of quick puffs before she came back into the room.

Later on we found a way to buy our own cigarettes. Clint's ice cream parlor had a cigarette machine in back. If no one was looking, you could sneak back there and drop in the coins and get your smokes.

Covington was a new school, but I was still the same kid. I was bored. I didn't take school seriously, even though my dad wanted me to. To inspire me, he gave me a leather briefcase to put my papers in and take to school. A leather briefcase! Can you imagine anything lamer than that? I was eleven years old. What did I want with a briefcase? So I found a bush where I could ditch the briefcase on my way to school and pick it up on my way home. Otherwise it would have been too embarrassing.

I don't remember having a favorite teacher. I didn't like any of them. I didn't like Mr. Pollock, the English teacher; or Mr. Proctor, the civics teacher; or Mr. Purdy, the PE teacher. I wasn't too keen on Mrs. Latham, the art teacher; or Mr. Christianson, the vice principal. I don't remember having a crush on any of my female teachers at Covington, either.

But I did have a crush on Janet Hammond. She lived in the house at the end of our street. My room looked down over her backyard. Unfortunately it didn't look down on *her*.

I thought about Janet a lot. I used to dream about being married to her. I used to dream about lying awake next to her at night or first thing in the morning—in bed, next to my wife. We were married, and we were happy. I wanted to have that feeling. I was so lonely all the time. I didn't have anyone special, just for me. So I dreamed about that. I would be married, and I'd never feel lonely anymore. I was thinking about getting away from Lou, I guess, and about getting away from home. I'd have my own house, and my own wife, and my own life. I'd be okay.

Sex was included in those daydreams. I had started to have sexual thoughts. And by junior high school I started noticing girls, big time. I noticed which ones had nice breasts, or nice rumps. I liked girls in short skirts—in those days, girls were not allowed to wear pants to school—and I loved their hairdos. I liked beehive hairdos, and hair that was teased out.

Girl watching didn't keep me out of trouble. It gave me something to daydream about, but between daydreams I got bored. And when I was bored, I got into trouble.

In wood shop in the seventh grade, I started out okay. I made a pair of salt-and-pepper shakers. But then I was fooling around with a chisel one day and I cut myself. The teacher got mad and wanted to know how I did it. He had just told us that day not to play around with the chisels. So I knew I couldn't tell him the truth. Instead, I lied and told him I had injured myself on the band saw.

That was a stupid excuse. He had already told us the band saw was strictly off-limits. We weren't allowed to be anywhere near it. So I got thrown out of wood shop, and I had to attend home economics. That wasn't so bad—it was all girls—but it was kind of embarrassing.

There were other incidents. I stole switchblade knives from lockers in the gymnasium, and got caught with them in my shoes.

But I didn't get caught for the most serious thing I did. One day I slipped into the girls' bathroom. It was empty. I had watched the door. I knew no one was in there. So I went in, and slipped into one of the stalls. I sat down and lit a cigarette, and waited. Girls started coming in. I think I had this idea that I would see things, and hear things, that would be sexy and exciting.

I didn't. I heard girls gossiping about stupid girl stuff, and I heard girls going to the bathroom. That's not what I was interested in. I wasn't kinky. I had healthy things in mind with girls. After a while I realized nothing good was going to happen. When the bathroom was empty again, I slipped back out.

But someone saw me, and reported me. I got called in and

questioned. Of course I denied it. And since no one had actually caught me, or even seen me, *in* the girls' bathroom, they couldn't really do anything to me. But I'm sure it went into my files. Did Lou and my dad ever know about it? I don't think so. If Lou had been aware of it, she would certainly have used it against me. She never mentioned it.

Things were bad at school. They were no better at home. I knew I was driving Lou crazy, and she was driving me crazy, too.

What I didn't know was that Lou had decided to do something about the problem. She had already spent a lot of time that fall visiting with doctors—talking about me, and trying to figure out what to do with me.

Sometime around 1958 or 1959, Lou had started taking classes at Foothill College, the local junior college in Mountain View. She had decided to become a medical assistant. What she learned in her classes started giving her ideas about what was wrong with me.

Brian remembers that she'd come home from school and tell him her theories. One of his jobs in the house was helping Lou wash and dry the dinner dishes. While they stood at the sink, she'd tell him her ideas. One of the first ones was that I had an extra chromosome. She told Brian there was something wrong with my brain.

Brian, even then, knew I wasn't retarded, or crazy. He did say that it seemed like I was always trying to get attention, and that my behavior was sometimes bizarre. He said I didn't take care of myself, and didn't care how I dressed or looked. He knew this bothered Lou. But he knew I wasn't sick, or crazy.

Lou didn't see it that way. She thought there was something wrong with me. She was determined to find out what it was and fix it.

Like I said before, Lou ran a tight ship. She was tough. She wasn't a quitter. She was probably what you'd call a control freak today. She wanted things her way. She *insisted* on having things her way.

But with me, she couldn't get her way. I was impossible to control. I was always in trouble at school and at home. I was big, and I had a lot of energy, and I made a lot of noise. If you ask me, I was just a kid. I was doing pretty much what kids that age do. But with me there was just a lot *more* kid stuff than there is with most kids. With me, it was all the time.

Lou was determined to make me act right. So she started talking with doctors, and taking me to see doctors.

I don't remember much about all that. I know that she had consulted with psychiatrists or psychologists before, because years later I saw some paperwork on it. She took me to a University of California clinic when I was seven, which I don't remember. She spoke to a Mr. Beal at the Family Services Department in Palo Alto, and spoke to someone at the Children's Health Council when I was nine or ten, which I also don't remember. When those visits ended, either the doctors weren't interested in me or she wasn't interested in them, I don't know which. And when she didn't get what she wanted from them, she started consulting with psychiatrists.

According to some of the doctors' notes and from what my dad told me later, Lou met with six psychiatrists during the spring and summer of 1960. She wanted to know what was wrong with me and what she should do about it.

But all six of the psychiatrists, I found out later, said my behavior was normal. Four of them even said the problem in the house was with *her*. They said *she* was the one who could benefit from treatment. Years later, Brian's wife told him that Lou had complained about this—that she had seen all those psychiatrists to get treatment for Howard, and some of them had said *she* was the problem. Could you believe the nerve of those doctors?

That wasn't the answer she was looking for. I'm sure it made her furious, too. So she kept looking for a doctor who would agree with her.

Sometime that fall, someone referred her to a doctor named Walter Freeman.

Chapter 5

Dr. Freeman

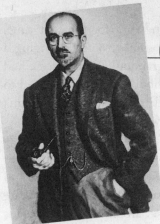

Walter Freeman was a nice looking, well educated, upper-class sort of guy. He was born in Philadelphia, one of seven children, into a family that traced its roots back to the Mayflower. (According to Freeman's biography, the excellent *The Lobotomist* by Jack El-Hai, one ancestor got drunk and fell *off* the Mayflower, and was saved by a boat hook.) Freeman's grandfather was a surgeon who had operated on President Grover Cleveland, and who became the first American surgeon to remove a brain tumor. (He did it with his fingers, without benefit of X-rays, in an operating theater that had no electric lighting. The patient lived another thirty years.) Freeman's father was a gifted surgeon as well.

Freeman grew up surrounded by money. He was tutored in dancing and riding, and cared for by a governess who spoke French, German, and Spanish. As a boy, he was called "Little Walter Wonder Why," because he was curious about everything.

His father was cold and strict. When Walter got in trouble at school, his father took out a leather whip—and beat *himself* with it for being a bad father. When Walter was given a gold coin for winning a prize at church, his father praised him—and then made him put the gold coin in the collection plate.

Freeman's mother was strict, too. Freeman later said that he admired her, but he never loved her.

Freeman attended Yale, where he was a dandy and dressed

strangely. A friend remembered meeting him for the first time. Freeman was wearing a wide Mexican sombrero and swinging a cane. He studied poetry, and used his grandfather's limousine and driver to take him and his friends to school dances. He decided to study medicine as a senior, and after Yale enrolled at Pennsylvania Medical School. He became fascinated with the brain.

After medical school, Freeman left America to study neurology and psychiatry at universities in Europe. He visited asylums in London and Paris, and worked with psychiatrists in Vienna and Rome. He came home depressed because he saw no real treatment for the insane. He wrote, "I looked around at the hundreds of patients and thought, 'What a waste.'" When he came back to America he opened a private practice and joined the faculty of George Washington University as a professor of neurology.

It was an exciting time in neurology. Millions of servicemen had been wounded in World War I and returned to England, Germany, France, and the United States with brain damage. In earlier wars, because there was no penicillin, soldiers like that would have died from their wounds. Now many of them came home alive, but brain-damaged. So scientists had this gigantic group of wounded men to study.

At the same time, there were huge advances in the new field of psychotherapy. Sigmund Freud had published his groundbreaking theories on the workings of human emotions. Those theories were beginning to find widespread acceptance.

But Freeman wasn't interested in Freud or psychoanalysis. He thought that approach could actually be dangerous: "When we realize, really get to know what stinkers we are, it takes only a little depression to tip the scales in favor of suicide," he wrote. Freeman believed instead that there were biological explanations for depression and schizophrenia, and that there had to be surgical treatments for them.

Over the next decade, attached to George Washington University, and working with George Washington Hospital and St. Elizabeth's Hospital, Freeman experimented on mental patients with a variety of radical new treatments. He subjected them to massive doses of insulin and the stimulant drug Metrazol, or hit them with giant volts of electroshock.

As a doctor he wasn't very successful. But as a teacher he was a big hit. His university lectures were like vaudeville shows, and drew huge audiences of medical students. Among other things, Freeman liked to write notes on the blackboard using both hands simultaneously.

He had a great sense of humor—even if it was sometimes a little weird. When he was a young doctor, he was asked to treat a young man whose girlfriend had placed a gold ring around his you-know-what. The young man got excited. Then he couldn't get the ring *off* his you-know-what, which started to turn blue. Freeman had the ring cut off, but then told the young man it would have to be kept as a "specimen." Freeman had the ring repaired and engraved. He wore it for years afterward, hanging from his watch chain, using it as a conversation starter.

Other doctors at the time were using many strange methods to treat patients who were depressed or mentally ill. Psychiatrists used electrotherapy, where they ran varying amounts of electricity through people's brains and bodies. They used hydrotherapy, where they gave their patients baths, douches, wet packs, steam, spritzers, and shots from hoses. Most of these were with cool or cold water, but another doctor used heat—hot baths, hot air, infrared lightbulb cabinets, and electric "mummy bags." A German psychiatrist developed something called the "electric shower." The patient was fitted into a helmet that gave his brain a "shower" of electricity.

One doctor used something called the "rest cure." That involved "isolation from family, quiet, diet, and massage." Another doctor used "sleep therapy." He would induce a deep sleep, almost a coma, and keep the patient there—for four to six weeks!

Some of the treatments were brutal. With hydrotherapy, doctors sometimes packed their patients in ice water, hoping that the freezing temperature would shock them into recovery. The insulin and Metrazol "therapies" caused such violent convulsions that patients broke their arms, legs, hips, and even *jaws*.

Some of the treatments seem just plain crazy now. One nut believed all mental illness was caused by infections. He said all psychotic patients had infected teeth. He started his campaign against mental infection by having all his patients' infected teeth removed. Then he decided to go further, and have all the other teeth removed, too. Then he started in on their tonsils. He was quoted at the time as saying that if all children had their tonsils removed, mental illness could be eliminated in a single generation. When the tonsillectomies didn't solve the problem, he started removing the colon, the cervix, and the uterus. He didn't cure any mental illness, but 30 percent of his patients were killed by the surgeries. He sounds like a guy who should have been locked up himself. Instead, he was the director of the New Jersey State Hospital in Trenton.

These doctors weren't just doing experiments in dark basements somewhere, hidden from the American Medical Association, or from the public eye. They were the subjects of articles in magazines and newspapers that applauded their efforts. *Time, Newsweek, Scientific American, Science Digest,* and *Reader's Digest* all published stories about the success rates of doctors working with insulin, hydrotherapy, and electrotherapy. (Most of them left out the details, like the stuff about the broken legs and fractured jaws.)

In 1935, visiting London, Freeman witnessed a presentation on chimpanzees whose frontal lobes had been operated on. No one knew why exactly, but the monkeys all became passive and subdued after the operation.

Another doctor attending the presentation was a Portuguese neurologist named Egas Moniz. He returned to Lisbon, and in late 1935 began performing similar frontal lobe experiments on human beings. Moniz called the process "psychosurgery." He drilled holes in his patients' heads, and made cuts in their frontal lobes, using a tool he called a "leucotome." He called the procedure itself a "leucotomy."

Moniz believed this was a promising treatment for mental illness. He published a paper stating that patients suffering from severe anxiety or depression seemed to respond best. Patients suffering from schizophrenia, he said, didn't respond at all.

Freeman read about Moniz's experiments in a French medical journal, and decided this was the answer. He contacted the company that supplied Moniz's leucotomes and ordered some for himself.

When the instruments arrived, Freeman and his partner, a surgeon named James Watt, began practicing on cadaver brains from the George Washington Hospital morgue. Watt was surprised to find that the human brain had the consistency, under a knife, of "soft butter." Shortly after, Freeman performed his first leucotomy. He and Watt drilled six holes into the shaved head of a sixty-three-year-old Kansas woman who had insomnia and fits of hysteria. Freeman and Watt used a coring tool to sever the connections between the body of her brain and its frontal lobes. The last thing the patient said before the anesthesia took hold was, "Who is that man? What is he going to do to me? Tell him to go away. Oh, I don't want to see him." Then she screamed and passed out.

The doctors said the surgery was a success. The patient lived only another five years, but Freeman said they were the happiest years of her life.

Over the next six weeks they did five more surgeries. After the first or second, Freeman proposed changing the name of the procedure from leucotomy to lobotomy. A month later, Freeman presented his findings at a psychiatry conference in Baltimore. In all of his patients, Freeman told his audience, there had been "worry, apprehension, anxiety, insomnia, and nervous tension." Now the patients were "more placid, content, and more easily cared for by their relatives."

He didn't tell his audience that his first patient, that Kansas woman, was comatose for a week after her surgery. For a week after that she couldn't speak, and for a week after that couldn't say her own name. A month later, she could recite the days of the week. Freeman reported that her "symptoms" were all gone. She wasn't hysterical, or frightened. She was looking forward to going home, he said.

Later, when asked about patients whose brains appeared to be damaged by the surgery, Freeman had this optimistic spin: "Maybe it will be shown that a mentally ill patient can think more clearly and constructively with less brain in actual operation."

Freeman started, with his first surgery, not quite telling the whole truth about his patients. He would continue to do this for the rest of his career. He often visited patients after their surgeries and pronounced them "cured" or "improved" because their worst symptoms had disappeared. But he made these visits four or five days after the surgery, when they were still barely conscious. Many of them would experience a complete return of their anxiety, or their hysteria, or their depression, but Freeman wouldn't know that, or wouldn't make note of it in his published papers or presentations at medical conventions.

Encouraged by the Kansas woman's surgery, Freeman and Watt conducted many more prefrontal lobotomies. In that early period, Freeman's statistics said that out of his first 623 surgeries, 52 percent of the patients received "good" results, 32 percent received "fair" results, and 13 percent received "poor" results. The remaining 3 percent died, but they weren't included in the "poor" results category. Freeman would later get closer to the truth when he admitted that his fatality rate was almost 15 percent.

The surgeries sometimes went badly. A Washington, D.C., police officer hemorrhaged after his lobotomy and became a vegetable. Leucotomes broke off in patients' heads. One patient died on the operating table when Freeman stopped, mid-surgery, to take a photograph.

This was part of Freeman's routine. He would always stop twice in the middle of the procedure to take his pictures. He'd stop once after he administered the electroshock, to take a "before" photo. He'd stop again in the middle of the lobotomy itself, to get a "during" photo. He'd sometimes take an "after" picture, too.

Later in his career, after another patient died during the photography session, Freeman started asking an assistant to hold the leucotomes for the "during" photograph, or he'd hold them himself and have someone else take the picture. But he never stopped documenting the procedure this way.

Many of Freeman's patients were so damaged by the surgery that they needed to be taught how to eat and use the bathroom again. Some never recovered. One of Freeman's most famous patients was Rosemary Kennedy, sister of future president John F. Kennedy. Rosemary was born slightly retarded, but she lived an almost normal life until she was twenty-three. Then Freeman went to work on her. He performed a prefrontal lobotomy in 1941. Rosemary wound up in a Wisconsin mental hospital, where she stayed until her death more than sixty years later.

Another famous lobotomy patient—but not one of Freeman's—was the actress Frances Farmer. She was a troubled woman but a great talent and a great beauty when she was hospitalized in Washington State for schizophrenia. She never acted again.

And she may never have had a lobotomy at all. The movie about her life, *Frances,* which was based on a book about her life, said she did. But I've read that her biographer admitted that he fictionalized many parts of her life. There is no record of her undergoing a lobotomy during her time as a mental patient.

The funny thing is, during all these surgeries, no one really knew why the lobotomies were successful. They only knew that for some reason interrupting the flow of energy in the brain seemed to interrupt the progression of anxiety or depression. They didn't know why. And they didn't know why it worked in some patients and not in others.

In an attempt to learn more about what happened during a lobotomy, Freeman tried performing them with the patient wide awake, under local anesthesia. During one of these procedures, Freeman asked the patient, while cutting his brain tissue, what was going through his mind. "A knife," the patient said. Freeman told this story with pleasure for years.

Many in the medical community weren't convinced that Freeman and Watt were on the right track. When Freeman asked William White, superintendent at Washington's St. Elizabeth's Hospital, for permission to conduct lobotomies there, he was told, "It will be a hell of a long time before I let you operate on any of *my* patients."

White had several objections. One of them, he said, was that mental patients often were not competent to agree to the surgery. They didn't understand what they were agreeing *to*. And the relatives who could agree to the surgery on their behalf didn't always have the patients' best interests at heart. "These sick people cause them a lot of trouble," White told Freeman. "In the back of their heads . . . relatives not infrequently desire the death of patients in hospitals."

Another colleague protested, when Freeman presented a paper on his first surgeries, "This is not an operation but a mutilation." He pointed out that many of the great men and women of history had suffered from depression, but still made enormous contributions to science and the arts. He asked Freeman, "What will be left of the musician or the artist when the frontal lobe is mutilated?"

Freeman got a mixed reaction from the medical community, but he always impressed the media. He was a real showman, and he courted the press. He often called reporters a day or two before he was going to make a presentation at a medical convention and asked them, "Do you want to see history made?" His partner, Watt, complained that Freeman was "like a barker at a carnival." On the medical convention floor, Freeman would set up a booth and use a clicker to attract a crowd. Then he'd begin talking about the lobotomy like it was some snappy new kitchen appliance.

He even had reporters attend lobotomies, and showed off for them while conducting the surgeries. One time, to demonstrate the simplicity of the procedure, he replaced the standard operating-room hammer with a wooden carpenter's mallet. Sometimes he performed a simultaneous two-handed lobotomy, severing both lobes at the same time with a flourish—just like he had impressed his students by using two hands to write on the board at the same time.

The news coverage was universally positive. Freeman's lobotomy was celebrated with headlines like PSYCHOSURGERY CURED ME, WIZARDRY OF SURGERY RESTORES SANITY TO FIFTY RAVING MANIACS, and NO WORSE THAN REMOVING A TOOTH.

This wasn't the tabloids. The *New York Times* ran a story applauding Freeman's success rate, which their reporter put at 65 percent, under the headline FIND NEW SURGERY AIDS MENTAL CASES.

Freeman's lobotomy might have gotten popular without the support of the press. America's hospitals were flooded with mental patients. By the late 1940s, there were more than a million mental cases in hospitals or asylums. More than 55 percent of all patients in American hospitals were mental cases. One study reported that the population of mental patients in American hospitals was growing by 80 percent a year.

There was no real treatment for these people. They were often drugged, shackled, kept in straitjackets, or locked in rubber rooms. Doctors were able to keep them from harming themselves or others, but they had a cure rate of about zero.

Besides, keeping them in hospitals was expensive. Freeman offered a solution. His motto was "Lobotomy gets them home!" Directors of mental institutions heard that loud and clear. One of Freeman's colleagues said that a procedure that would send 10 percent of mental patients home would save the American taxpayer $1 million a day. Freeman claimed a success rate well above 10 percent. Most hospitals and institutions welcomed him and his lobotomy.

Freeman was sort of like the Henry Ford of psychosurgery. He didn't invent the procedure, but he turned it into an assembly-line process, streamlining it so it could be done more efficiently, more cheaply, more quickly, and on more patients.

By the early 1940s Freeman was a successful doctor. He was famous. He had married and produced a big family. He and his wife, Marjorie, had six children, one girl and five boys. Freeman liked family vacations. Every summer he'd take his family on long drives to lakes and rivers for hikes or camping expeditions. He might have just enjoyed life and coasted on his reputation as the American father of the prefrontal lobotomy. But he was ambitious.

In the early 1940s Freeman heard about an Italian surgeon who was trying to refine the prefrontal lobotomy by entering the brain without drilling or cutting the skull, through the thin bone at the back of the eye socket—known as the orbit. Freeman read up on this procedure, and in early 1946 conducted America's first transorbital lobotomy. He used an ice pick on his first patient. (He saved the ice pick. It's in Washington, D.C., with his archives. It says "Uline Ice Company" on the handle.)

The patient's name was Sally Ellen Ionesco. She was twenty-nine, and she had suffered years of depression and manic behavior. She sometimes became violent with her young daughter, or with herself, and had tried to jump out a window.

Freeman went into her brain through the eye socket on one side, and had her come back a week later to do the other side.

The surgery was apparently successful. After a rough period of adjustment, the patient found that her violent outbursts were gone. "It was like, 'Thank God, it's over,'" her daughter later told Freeman's biographer. "There was peace." Although she required a private nurse for a while, Sally Ellen Ionesco gradually became well enough to take care of her daughter, to help her husband in the family business, and later to be licensed as a practical nurse and get work as a nanny.

To Freeman, the new transorbital technique represented an incredible improvement. Without cutting and drilling, lobotomies could be done in doctors' offices. There would be no surgeon, no anesthesiologist, no hospital stay, and almost no recovery time. Freeman thought he could send his patients home an hour after the procedure.

He began doing lobotomies in his office. He stretched the patients out on a table, knocked them out using electroshock, punctured the skull using his Uline ice pick, and swung the ice pick back and forth across their frontal lobes. He waited for the bleeding to stop, then sent the patient home, sometimes in a taxi cab.

When nothing went wrong, the patients were left with no visible damage except for a pair of very blackened eyes. Freeman was funny about this—in an insensitive way. He said, "I usually asked the family to provide the patient with sunglasses rather than explanations."

But things did go wrong. The fourth transorbital patient hemorrhaged during the procedure. Freeman couldn't stop the bleeding. The patient was rushed to a hospital and saved, but suffered from epileptic fits for the rest of his life, which he spent selling newspapers on a street corner.

On another occasion, Freeman stopped mid-surgery to set up the camera and document the procedure. For some reason the ice pick began to slide down into the patient's brain. He died without ever regaining consciousness.

James Watt refused to assist with the transorbital procedure, which he said was unprofessional and unsafe. Other colleagues agreed. A hospital medical director, one of Freeman's earlier supporters, wrote to him and said, "What are these terrible things I hear about you doing lobotomies in your office with an ice pick? Why not use a shotgun? It would be quicker!"

Freeman was not bothered by these reactions. He was sure he had found a fast, cheap, and effective way to treat hopeless mental patients. To prove it, he began touring the country and visiting mental institutions. He would perform transorbital lobotomies and, in the process, teach the resident psychiatrists how to do the operation themselves.

He worked hard at it, and he did it practically for free. He charged large institutions twenty-five dollars a patient to perform the lobotomy at a time when, as a private physician, he could have charged thousands. In one year he visited hospitals in seventeen states, and also made presentations in Canada, Puerto Rico, and South America. On one five-week driving tour of America, he visited eight states and performed 111 lobotomies.

He made these tours driving a specially outfitted car that he called "The Lobotomobile." The first one was a custom-fitted

Lincoln Continental. Later he would drive a van. Whatever the model was, he carried in it photographic equipment, to make records of the surgeries and the patients, a card catalog of patients' records, a portable electroshock machine, a Dictaphone for taking notes while he drove, and his surgical instruments.

One summer he logged 11,000 miles in his Lobotomobile. He kept a diary of his work. The entries alone make you tired.

> 29 June, Little Rock, Arkansas, 4 patients
> 30 June, Rusk, Texas, 10 patients
> 1 July, Terrell, Texas, 7 patients
> 2 July, Wichita Falls, Texas, 3 patients
> 9 July, Patton, California, 5 patients
> 14 July, Berkeley, California, 3 patients

State hospitals tended to be more willing to try the treatment than private ones, because state hospitals were overcrowded and underfunded and would do almost anything to send a few patients home. The Stockton State Hospital in California had more than 4,000 patients when it started doing lobotomies, and between 1947 and 1954 did 232 of them. Most of the lobotomy patients were women. The author Joel Braslow, in his book *Mental Ills and Bodily Cures,* said almost the same number of patients died from the operation as were sent home by it—21 percent were killed, and 23 percent were cured.

Freeman was ready to do the surgery whenever, wherever. One of his surgical assistants—Jonathan Williams, who replaced James Watt after Watt refused to go along with Freeman's plan to do lobotomies in his office, without a surgeon present—later told a story about a patient who had been brought to Freeman for a lobotomy. The day before the surgery, though, he'd gotten cold feet and refused to go through with the operation. He locked himself in his hotel room. Freeman, contacted by the patient's family, drove to the hotel and convinced the patient to let him in. Using a portable electroshock machine he had designed and built for himself, he administered a few volts to the patient to calm him down. According to Williams, "The patient was . . . held down on the floor while Freeman administered the shock. It then occurred to him that since the patient was already unconscious, and he had a set of leucotomes in his pocket, he might as well do the transorbital lobotomy then and there, which he did."

Williams said that, over time, the portable electroshock device began to fall apart. First the dial for setting the voltage broke. Then the timer broke. In the end, Freeman would simply connect the patient to the machine, plug it in, and flip the switch—relying on his own instincts to guess how much juice was going into the patient, and how long to leave it running.

There's all kinds of evidence that Freeman did not have much patience for standard medical practice, and that he preferred to get right to work without taking the ordinary precautions. Sometimes this resulted in Freeman breaking off the ends of the leucotomes while they were still in the patient's skull. On more than one occasion, Williams had to open the skull the old-fashioned way and surgically remove two or three inches of broken-off steel from behind the eye sockets, cleaning up after Freeman had made a mess.

Williams said that Freeman hated wasting time on creating a sterile environment for the surgery. He wasn't worried about what he called "all that germ crap," Williams said. "I often had to assert myself, insisting, 'Walter, at least let me drape the patient.' "

Freeman's cross-country campaigns spread the lobotomy far and wide, and fast. Dozens of doctors trained by Freeman began performing their own surgeries. There are no official numbers on this, but some estimates say Freeman did more than 5,000 lobotomies in his career. People taught by him may have done 40,000 more.

Freeman's lobotomy began falling out of favor. By the early 1950s it was still a common surgery, but its long-term benefits were beginning to be questionable. Then, in 1954, the Food and Drug

Administration approved use of the chemical compound chlorpro-mazine, which was sold under the name Thorazine. Freeman dis-missed it as "chemical lobotomy," and thought it was inefficient. The patient would have to continue taking the drug forever, while the lobotomy required one procedure for life. But the medical com-munity embraced Thorazine, and many other drugs developed af-terward. They were easy to administer, required no training to administer, didn't have fatal side effects, and could be stopped at any time without permanent damage.

The lobotomy passed into literature and legend—Ken Kesey's *One Flew Over the Cuckoo's Nest*, and the bar joke "I'd rather have a bottle in front of me than a frontal lobotomy"—and became in-creasingly unpopular as a medical procedure. (I've heard it was Tom Waits who made up the line about the bottle. Kesey had a job at a mental hospital—maybe the Veterans Administration hospital in Palo Alto—where he saw firsthand the results of lobotomy and other mistreatment.)

The lobotomy may have become passé, but Walter Freeman never stopped believing in it, promoting it, or performing it.

In 1954, he left Washington, D.C., for the West Coast. He was fifty-eight. It was clear to him that he could go no further profes-sionally in the medical establishment. His work was too controver-sial for him to ever be head of the American Medical Association or run a major psychiatric institution. Besides, he had always hated the weather—too cold in winter, too muggy in summer. He moved to California.

There were personal reasons, too. Two of his children had fin-ished their university educations, married, and settled in the Bay Area. And in California he could be closer to the places he loved to walk and hike—Yosemite, the Sierras, the Grand Canyon.

In addition, his wife was a heavy drinker, and that had become a problem. A fresh start for him would be a fresh start for her, too.

Freeman, being Freeman, didn't just move. He moved with *style*. He knew he wanted to live somewhere around Palo Alto, but he wasn't sure which community was best for him. So he hired a private plane, and spent half a day having a pilot fly him over the area. Some guys would've just looked at a map and talked to some real estate agents. Not Freeman. By the end of the day, he settled on green, leafy, high-class Los Altos. He and his wife bought a house in the foothills.

Freeman was sort of a celebrity in the medical world, and he was welcomed by the local medical community. But his lobotomy was not. Freeman set up offices at 15 Main Street, right in central Los Altos, but no hospital in Los Altos would allow him to operate. He had to go all the way to Doctors General Hospital, on the outskirts of San Jose, to perform his procedure.

This was more than a medical decision. Los Altos was a *nice* place. It wasn't supposed to have problems like mental illness. Los Altos had manicured gardens and clean sidewalks and showcase homes. It didn't have crazy people. Even though Freeman was an educated and cultured man, erudite and charming, the people of Los Altos probably thought his medical procedure was low-rent and tacky. It was for people in loony bins, and there weren't any loony bins in Los Altos. The local attitude was, "We just don't *do* lobotomies here."

I don't think my stepmother was shopping for a lobotomy the first time she met Freeman. But she was fed up with me, that was certain.

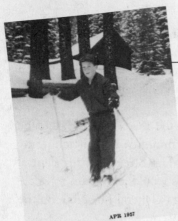

APR 1957

Chapter 6

DULLY, Howard
(F: Rodney L.)

On October 5, 1960, Lou had her first meeting with Dr. Freeman. Freeman's notes from the first session read like this:

Mrs. Dully came in to talk about her step-son who is now 12 years old and in the 7th grade. There are four other boys in the family, two of hers, aged 17 and 12, another of his, aged 9, and a four-year-old that belongs to both of them. Mrs. Dully's first husband was an alcoholic who impoverished her, ran off with a girlfriend who took him for a ride and divorced him, and he doesn't seem to enter the picture. Mrs. Dully's boys are good-natured and well behaved. Howard's mother had a third child before she died of cancer; this child was adopted and turned out to be a mental defective and, I believe, is in an institution and not expected to live beyond puberty. Mr. Dully is a teacher of the 6th and 7th grades in the Hillview School for the last six or seven years while Mrs. Dully didn't finish high school. She got to know Mr. Dully shortly after he was widowed when Howard was about five years old; she did some sewing and washing and commiserating, and according to Mrs. Dully, her husband is the best husband imaginable, kind, considerate, a good provider, willing to do without, sharing her problems, with no difficulties in regard to religion, money or politics, but he can't see anything wrong with Howard, and that's where they disagree most particularly.

Freeman was a great keeper of notes. I don't know if he wrote them, or dictated them to a secretary, or used that tape recorder he carried around in the Lobotomobile. But he kept close notes. The first meeting generated two full pages, single-spaced. The whole file on me runs about thirty pages. Each page is topped with the patient's name—it doesn't mention Lou; it's DULLY, Howard (F: Rodney L.)—address and phone number, and date. The referring doctor's name, Marazzo, appears on every page, too.

Freeman didn't write much about what he thought. But he wrote a lot about what other people said. Unlike the psychiatrists Lou had already seen, Freeman didn't seem interested in talking to her about *her*. The file was about me. In fact, the first interview with Lou read like testimony in a murder trial. Freeman even referred to it as "the articles of indictment."

The first time Mrs. Dully saw the boy she thought he was a spastic because of his awkward swing of the arms in walking and a peculiar gait. He seems to have poor muscular control but he's good at many of the athletic games at school. He dislikes to work with his hands; he doesn't build. His younger brother, Bryan [Freeman wrote it like that] likes to build houses, walls, castles of blocks, and Howard knocks them down, throws the blocks at the walls and pounds Bryan on the head with them. He objects to going to bed but then sleeps well. He watches his chances and is clever at stealing but always leaves something behind to show what he's done. If it's a banana, he throws the peel at the window; if it's a candy bar, he leaves the wrapper around someplace, and hides things in such obvious places as behind the bureau and under the bed. He doesn't play with toys, rather he uses them as weapons or is destructive with them. There's a dog in the home and he teases the dog until it becomes excited and then he punishes the dog for getting excited. He scowls and frowns if the TV is turned on to some other program than what he likes, which is mostly blood and thunder. He does a good deal of daydreaming and when asked about it, he says: "I don't know." He is defiant at

times—"You tell me to do this, and I'll do that." He has a vicious
expression on his face some of the time.

Freeman called the indictment "sufficiently impressive." Suffi-
cient for *what*? To qualify me as a patient for counseling? For a lobotomy? It's not clear from Freeman's notes what he made of Lou
or her "indictment."

The second page got a little more intense.

When [Howard] and his step-brother, who are both about the
same age, were dressed for school he didn't want to wear the new
clothes but wore his jeans and shirts often ragged, puts a sweater
on on the hottest days and goes without an undershirt on a chilly
one; he turns the room lights on when there's broad sunlight out-
side and strains his eyes to see in the dark when it comes; he hates
to wash. Mrs. Dully had to put him on the toilet until he was
6 years old and had to bathe him until he was 8. He used to have
rather severe nosebleeds, maybe from picking, but even when
blood was smeared on his face and pillow he didn't tell about it
and didn't seem to realize or acknowledge anything wrong. He
still sometimes defecates in his pants or in bed or on the floor, or
may wrap up a turd and hide it in the drawer; recently he uri-
nated on the wall of his room; at another time he dribbled from
his room all the way to the bathroom; used toilet paper can be
found in his closet or in his bed or in the tub.

Mrs. Dully wanted to take Howard again to Family Service.
But her husband objected and will probably object to coming to
the office and giving his side of the picture. She thinks he is very
proud and that he denies trouble rather than face it. He did have
to clean up one mess after Howard had urinated on the floor so
that it went through the ceiling below.

The only peace of mind that Mrs. Dully has at the present
time is when Mr. Orville Black, who is a janitor, takes Howard
each Sunday for the past couple of months and is apparently able

to relate to him. I asked Mrs. Dully to have Mr. Black come in
and tell me his experiences with the boy on Sundays.

> *From her story, it would seem to be childhood schizophrenia,*
and this is rather borne out by some drawings which she found
stashed away in his closet.

Those were the notes from Lou's first visit. Could any of it be true? I'm sure I didn't wash well enough to satisfy Lou. I might have stained my underpants, or dribbled on my way to the toilet. I'm sure I blew my nose and dropped the tissue on the floor. But, wrapping up a turd and hiding it? Come on!

The truest thing Lou said was that my father would object to seeing Freeman. I wasn't part of any discussion about it, but my little brother Brian remembered terrible arguments about me going on at home. My father thought I was fine. Lou thought I was crazy. They screamed at each other, Brian said, using words so ugly that he ran and hid in his room.

But my father's resistance didn't stop Lou, or Freeman. Three days later he had a visit from Orville Black. Freeman's notes from the meeting told a different story from the one he got from Lou.

Mr. Black is a middle-aged man with iron-grey hair. I gather
from Mr. Black that Mrs. Dully is perpetually talking, admon-
ishing, correcting and getting worked up into a spasm, whereas
her husband is impatient, explosive, rather brutal, in fact, in the
way he won't let the boy speak for himself, and calls him numb-
skull, dimwit and other uncomplimentary names. Under Mr.
Black's rather serene directions Howard has not only looked after
himself, such as going and washing his hands, straightening
things out, but has been quite helpful at a church picnic where he
helped set the table and lay out things and also has shown polite-
ness and consideration of others. Recently, with a boy named Bob,
they were doing some miniature golf and Howard left Bob when
the latter showed lack of control in hitting the balls too hard and

making them bounce. Howard has even expressed a desire to go to Sunday school . . .

Mr. Black is much more than a janitor at school since he is the confidant of all the lonely boys that can get lost among 300 other boys. He takes pride in being "easy to talk to." He says that both Mr. and Mrs. Dully are attempting to tone down their criticism of Howard in the hope of getting a better response.

A list of typed topics appears to go with Freeman's notes from the meeting. Under the heading "Report of Mr. Black," someone typed things like "Shows frustration. Feels hemmed in. Has confidence in no one. Doubts he can please anyone or do anything right. Has mind of his own. Would like to be trusted. Would try to please anyone he could trust as a friend. Must be handled with positive but friendly attitude."

Four days later, Lou was back again. She admitted, according to the notes, "Howard did very well Saturday afternoon and Sunday when he was with Mr. Black," but said, "Sunday evening when he came back he reverted to his former behavior, has been unbelievably defiant, with a savage look on his face, and at times she is almost afraid that he will harm her or somebody else."

Freeman wrote that my dad was away for a few days but that "he might be the next person to contact." He also wrote that Lou wanted to bring in her sister, who "was of the opinion that it was step-mother trouble until about a year ago but has now changed her mind."

Freeman seemed to be looking forward to meeting them. "It should be an interesting family constellation," he concluded.

I wish I remember more about this period. It was October. The days were starting to get shorter, and cooler. The leaves were changing color and the trees were getting bare. The World Series was coming. Thanksgiving, Christmas, and my birthday weren't too far off.

But I don't remember much. I didn't know Lou was seeing Freeman. I didn't know she was talking about me with psychiatrists. I remember spending those Sundays with Uncle Orville. I remember Lou being mad at me all the time. I remember being called those kinds of names, by her and by my dad.

I remember, for some reason, sitting in the backyard on a little swing set we had there and singing to myself. I liked music, and I liked listening to music, and I often sang songs to myself. (Later on I would take up the guitar and develop the idea that I could be some kind of pop star.) I remember sitting in the backyard, swinging and singing softly to myself. The song was "Moments to Remember," by The Four Lads.

The lyrics are supposed to be sort of nostalgic. The song has nice harmonies and these sort of glockenspiel bells. The words say:

> *The New Year's Eve we did the town*
> *The day we tore the goal post down*
> *We will have these moments to remember*

I'd rock back and forth and sing to myself and the tears would roll down my cheeks. What was I crying about? I didn't go to college yet. I didn't miss those crazy college days and my old college pals. But I could relate to the sadness of the song.

Sometime during this period, Brian was pulled into the argument about me, and what to do with me. He was taken in by Lou to see Dr. Lopes, who for many years had been our pediatrician. When he got there, Dr. Lopes asked Lou to wait outside. He wanted to speak to Brian alone.

Lopes wanted to talk about me. He wanted to ask Brian questions about what was happening with me. He told Brian that my family was thinking about sending me away because of my behavior.

Brian broke down. He burst into tears. He told the doctor that he didn't want them to send me away. He wanted me to stay at home with him. He told the doctor there wasn't anything wrong with me.

Brian would have been about nine at the time. It was the end of his relationship with the pediatrician. He said later, "That's the last time I ever saw Dr. Lopes. The next time I got sick, I was taken to see Dr. Philips. I never saw Dr. Lopes again. Lou was shopping around for answers, and Dr. Lopes, after talking to me, had come to the wrong conclusion."

In spite of Lou's interest in getting me out of the house, and using Freeman to do it, the family was having financial difficulties, and Freeman was charging more than they could afford. There's a letter from that period, written in November, that Lou wrote to Freeman: "We hope you will accept this payment now and we shall make future payments until paid in full or up to date," Lou wrote. "If I find a buyer for my antique glassware you shall be paid much sooner."

It must have been serious if Lou was selling her antiques. But I guess she found the money somewhere, because the meetings with Freeman continued. The cast of characters increased, too.

Lou got her sister Virginia to come talk to Freeman. She had a lot to say, and I'm sure Lou wanted her to say it as soon as possible.

"Mrs. Dully came in with her sister, Mrs. Virginia Robinson, to discuss Howard," Freeman's notes said.

> Mrs. Robinson started off by saying that she has six children, one by a former marriage, Linda who is now 16, and who says that Howard gives her the creeps. He'll sneak up behind her without making any noise and seems to love to startle a person. He looks at one out of the corner of his eye. He seems to have a perverted sense of humor and will repeat something that isn't funny over and over. He forgets that he's supposed to do something and may come back three or four times from upstairs, where he's been told to get something, asking what it was. He seems to be in a fog. Mrs. Robinson considers him a tortured little soul and she pities him, but recognizes the aggravation.

Lou must have stayed on without Virginia, or maybe she continued her indictment with Virginia still there. Freeman's notes for that day went on:

Mrs. Dully had a talk with the teacher and the latter said that she has 160 pupils and 159 of them she can reach but she can't reach Howard; he won't bring his books to school and when scolded he couldn't seem to care less. However, at times he does so well that he'll get an A and the next time an F. Mrs. Dully says that Mr. Black considers Howard normal but "When Howard pulls some of that stuff I almost wanted to hit him right then and there." He says every child must have some fear, but that Howard seems to be afraid of everything.

Next to that, in pencil, was a handwritten word: "Why?" Good question. The next couple of entries offered some explanations.

Mrs. Dully reports that when Howard brought home one of his bad reports his father got mad at him and his mother had to control the father so he wouldn't abuse the boy; his father being a sixth grade teacher, he might have exercised better control.

Howard cries more easily than anybody either of these ladies knows. For instance, when the boys were making a racket Mrs. Dully told them all to go get out of the house, and when she looked out some time later Howard was way over at the end of the lot, all alone, and she went to him and tears were falling down his cheeks; she patiently explained that all the boys had been reproved and that he shouldn't take it too seriously.

Any doctor could guess from that report that I was a sensitive kid and that I was living in a difficult environment. He could probably not guess how bad it was. But Lou was filling his head with details: "Mrs. Dully left a number of other observations," Freeman wrote.

In one handwritten document, dated October 19, 1960, there was a long list of additional complaints. I don't know if the handwriting was Lou's, but the complaints were. And they were really ugly.

"Has monkey-like gestures and mannerisms—i.e., scratching head and body," the notes say. "Tires easily. Needs more sleep. Falls asleep easily in chair. Eyes bloodshot when tired. Not responsive. No appealing to him. Jekel [*sic*] and Hyde disposition."

The notes say I couldn't dress myself properly, that I got dirty all the time, that I was difficult to manage. But they all seemed like such petty complaints. "Won't move when told time is short. Doesn't use good judgment. Comprehension not good. Seems useless to convey reasons. Won't do homework."

There was also some evidence that, to me, seems like it might have been a red flag to any doctor or psychiatrist who was really listening. "Peeps through windows, whether inside or out," the notes said. "Facial muscles contract. But no twitch or tics. Shows inward suffering, but can't describe. Extreme state of agitation. Eyes shift in peculiar manner."

Those details make me sound like a kid under a huge amount of stress. And some of what she told Freeman makes Lou herself sound disturbed. Freeman's last notes from that day said:

Finally, she said that she's being plagued by dreams of Howard. In one of these, which keeps recurring, she wants to spank him but finds that she has no right arm, that it's just a weak little nub, and she interprets this as meaning that she'll never be able to spank him. Another time a dream recurred twice that she had her teeth all set to sink in to him and woke to find herself biting the pillow.

Freeman was not ready to make a recommendation. He wanted more information.

"I declined to give any statement until I've seen Howard," he wrote. "And said I would have to see Mr. Dully first."

Before he could meet with me or my dad, Freeman got a visit from Orville's wife, Evelyn. On October 21, he wrote,

Mrs. Black says that Rodney's mother [my dad's mom, my grandma Boo] was quite aggressive and that she rejected him almost completely so that when Rodney was about 6 years old he was put under the care of Mrs. Black who was quite a different person. "The only love Rodney ever had was mine." The Blacks had lived in a logging camp for some 17 years and Rodney spent several summers there. He never gave his love to his children and, as a result, his son Howard "does not know how to love. He can't speak up. Rodney is ruining Howard but he is afraid to talk to anybody. Rodney hushes Howard all the time. Howard seems to like to eat, just like his father did, and eat all the time, and Rodney has been heard to say to him, 'Well, God damn you, you've just eaten two hours ago. Why the Hell do you have to eat now?' " Mrs. Black says, "Like father, like son." She believes it is quite possible for both the Dullys to change their attitude toward Howard. She feels Howard is a much-maligned lad and that he only needs tender loving care to bring him out of his present state. She doesn't see anything wrong with him.

Three days later, Freeman had his first meeting with my father.

Mr. Dully came in for a talk about Howard, and says: "The whole family revolves around Howard." Mr. Dully is unwilling to say there's anything really wrong with Howard, that it may be either with himself or with Mrs. Dully. Nevertheless, he has no such trouble with the other children in the family. I inquired specifically about instances of precocity in Howard's case and his father remembered at the age of 2 he found a box of nuts, bolts, switches, wires and screws and a lot of electrical equipment; he took out each piece, examined it carefully, put it aside and after he was finished he put it all back again. Mr. Dully teaches the sixth grade at Hillview and has a lot of other youngsters to compare Howard to but he's unable to do so. He says when he loses his temper he really beats the boy in a cruel fashion, whereas he's never laid a hand on the other boys. Then Howard comes back and reproaches him, saying: "You tell me it's the family as a whole, but I'm the only one that gets it." This makes Mr. Dully try to restrain himself when Howard does something particularly infuriating. However, he has often caught the boy in a lie, recognizes he's a sneak, and was particularly disturbed the way Howard was falling down in his school work with social science and language, although he's doing well enough in mathematics. His performance is so variable as to be a constant source of puzzlement—for instance, the first time Mr. Dully took Howard skiing the boy did very well, and yet the next time he didn't do well at all. In spite of what Mrs. Dully says about his clumsiness, the boy can throw a ball well and run well. He doesn't seem to have any particular likes, mostly dislikes, as though he lives in fear all the time.

Two days later, on the afternoon of Wednesday, October 26, Freeman had his first meeting with *me*.

Freeman seemed at first like a kind, gentle, dapper man. He had a high forehead, a receding hairline, and a pointed goatee. He had round glasses and attentive eyes. He wore a suit and tie.

I liked him at once. He paid attention to me. First of all, he asked me questions about myself. He asked me what I liked to do, and what I didn't like, and why. He asked me what I thought about things, and how I felt about things. No one had ever asked me how I *felt* about things, but he did.

And, even more important, when he asked me a question he actually *listened* to the answer.

Freeman's office was in a little collection of doctors' and dentists' offices near the corner of Fremont and Mary. The place was very clean, and the grounds were very well manicured, and the office looked more like a businessman's office than a doctor's office. It was furnished in rich, brown leather. There was no medical equipment in it. There was hardly any paper in it.

Freeman was dressed nicely, in either a sport coat or a suit—not a doctor's coat. I'd never seen a psychiatrist or a neurologist before, so I didn't know whether this was normal, but I liked it. And I liked Freeman. He put me at ease. He had a soft voice and warm eyes. He smiled at me. I thought the goatee was cool, too. It made him look a little like a beatnik—like Dobie Gillis or Maynard G. Krebs.

Freeman wanted me to talk about Lou. He asked me whether I disliked her, and why. He wanted to know if I felt like hurting her. I was very open with him. I said that I didn't want to hurt her, but that I wanted to get *away* from her. I told him that she spanked me, and that I got the wrath of my father when he came home. I told him that it was hard for me to be in trouble all the time, and that it didn't seem fair.

He understood, or he acted like he did. Nothing seemed to faze him. He sat back. He listened. He took notes. Later—that visit, or another visit, I'm not sure—he gave me some inkblots to look at. I'd never seen any before, and I thought they were weird, and kind of neat. The pictures reminded me of bats and things. I saw women in some of them. I told Freeman that. He just smiled and took notes. I had no idea, of course, what he was writing down.

But this is what his notes said about our first visit:

Howard is a rather tall, slender, somewhat withdrawn type of individual. The first interview today was largely in the matter of getting acquainted. I spoke first of his interest in mechanical things and he began to talk about his bicycle and how the handlebars have been poorly adjusted; he was trying to do something about them. But he also spoke of recently patching a tire five times in one day, after which he got a new tire. But he likes his old bicycle, even though it's only a 26". He told about his paper route which brings him some $20 each month and he's saving up to get a record player, but he finds he spends his money, sometimes without too much thinking about it. He's helped his half-brother George on three occasions, yet this morning when he asked George *to help him wrap the papers in wax paper (there was a little shower) George refused, and I could see there was a good deal of resentment on Howard's part. We also talked about his interest in science. He's interested in diagrams and animals but he curled up his nose when it came to describing the dissection of a frog's stomach. When he had started, he talked fairly freely, said that when it's a question of being out on a hike he likes to get off the beaten path and go up the sides of hills, the dry-water courses and so on, but that when he goes with a crowd the leader insists on sticking to the well-worn paths and keeps him from climbing trees and doing other things he'd like to. He's been fishing only twice and caught fish only once so this is a phase to be opened. He goes around Lake Tahoe for a week in the summertime and sometimes in the winter, has done some skiing but no water skiing.*

I don't remember how the first visit ended, but when Lou told me I would have to see Freeman again, I was happy. I remember looking forward to it.

One week later, I was back in his office. Freeman took more notes:

Howard is rather evasive talking about things that go on in the home. He drew me a floor plan of the house. This was drawn fairly competently. He says that in the morning he gets out early and delivers his papers; he has a new bicycle now which seems to be fine; it has three speeds and good brakes so that he can get around the hills. He gets home in time for breakfast which consists of orange juice and cereal and toast, with once in a while an egg, but he seems to be satisfied with it, and after school he has some chores to do around the house which he doesn't talk much about. It seems that Mr. Dully is down for breakfast but he takes very little part in the family circle since, when he comes home, about all he does is to slump down in a chair in front of the TV or start reading. He has to go out three or four evenings a week. Howard is closest to George and Howard believes he gets more than his share of the punishment but says that George is cleverer at avoiding discovery and often gets by with things that he would be punished for. The school work seems difficult for Howard even tho' he does study he doesn't seem to recall things, and he does poorly on the tests. He was talking about the ancient Chinese civilization, which they are doing in Social Studies now; this doesn't seem to interest him at all. Nothing really seems to interest him. He gets to playing checkers and particularly chess with George and usually beats him. He doesn't mention much about Brian or the older brother. Things have to be more or less prodded out of him, and while not being evasive, he doesn't convey much information.

Another week later, on November 9, I was back. This time Freeman gave me a physical. He reported that I was sixty-two inches tall, weighed ninety-five pounds, and had pouches under my eyes and big hands and feet. He found everything about me normal—reflexes, "sensibility," blood pressure, and so on—but didn't have much else to say about me.

So, one more week after that, I was back again. It was almost like Freeman couldn't figure out what to do with me. On November 16, he wrote about me making the rounds on my paper route, about my apparent lack of interest in sports, about my skill at chess—"He can find very few people to play with him since he can lick his father and George without half trying." Freeman suggested I might want to go on a "ramble" in the Black Mountains with him. I said that Sundays were out because that was my time with Orville and Evelyn Black. I complained to Freeman a little about how I always seemed to get blamed no matter what went wrong. "They come down on him like a ton of bricks," Freeman wrote. But, he added, "Howard does not dwell on the fact that he is discriminated against . . ."

This must have been frustrating to Lou. She had found a doctor who seemed to listen to her, and who seemed to take her problems with me seriously. But he had seen me four times, and from his notes it would appear that the more time he spent with me the more normal he found me. He even wanted to take me hiking.

So Lou turned up the gas a little.

"Mrs. Dully came in for a talk about Howard. Things have gotten much worse during the past two or three months and she can barely endure it."

The date was November 30. It wasn't even two months since their first visit. They'd been talking the whole time. This new tone—about things getting much worse—was ominous.

> She has to keep the boys constantly separated in order to avoid something serious happening, and she now has to protect even the dog because Howard will pretend to pet the dog and at the same time twist the collar around so as to strangle the animal. Howard does sneaky little things, pinching and sticking pins in his little brother, and always seems to have the idea that everybody is against him.
>
> Mrs. Dully thinks that her husband sits down in front of the television and goes to sleep because he doesn't want to hear any of the problems that are so pressing. She feels she is unable to reach him because he just closes up. She thinks that maybe Howard's uncle, who is looking after the youngest brother, a mental defective, might be willing to take on Howard if Mr. Dully approves of this. I think it would be pretty much of a shame to wish Howard on anybody.

Freeman had heard enough. It was time for action. He told Lou that it was possible the children's ward at the Langley Porter Clinic—a famous neuropsychiatric institute attached to the University of California in San Francisco—might have room for me, or that someone from Children's Services might be able to help.

Freeman concluded that set of notes by saying, "Howard has an extremely individualistic approach to things, and if any attempt is made to control him he takes it personally and thinks it's all part of the persecution that is constantly going on."

But nothing would really fix me, Freeman said, except a lobotomy.

"I explained to Mrs. Dully," Freeman said in his notes, "that Howard was unapproachable by psychotherapy since I believed him to be essentially a schizophrenic, and that the family should consider the possibility of changing Howard's personality by means of transorbital lobotomy. Mrs. Dully said it was up to her husband, that I would have to talk with him and explain the impossible situation that was arising in the home and make it stick."

It had taken less than two months, and four visits from Lou, and four visits with me, to convince Dr. Freeman that a transorbital lobotomy was the only answer to our family's problems. That's how easily the decision was made. Lou told Freeman it was up to my dad. Freeman told Lou he might confer with Dr. Kirk McGuire, a family friend who was the namesake of my baby brother, and get him on the team.

The really sad part is that this decision took place on November 30, 1960: It was my twelfth birthday. Lou went home that evening to tell my father what he had to do.

The following day, my dad was in Freeman's office. December 1, 1960, was a Thursday. My dad had to take time off work—either from teaching, from Whitecliff Market, or from Kodak—to make the appointment. He must have understood it was serious.

If not, Freeman set him straight right away.

Mr. Dully came in for a review of the situation, and I gave it as my opinion that Howard was a schizophrenic and that unless something was done pretty promptly I thought the situation would be irreversible. Mr. Dully gave me two bits of new information; in the first place, [Howard] was very devoted to his own mother and never seemed to get along with his step-mother, although she tried to win him over. In the second place, Howard has been heard repeatedly talking to himself and Mr. Dully has tended to disregard this as he has the other things, but when it's

called to his attention he recognizes that possibly it is serious. He
will talk the matter over with Mrs. Dully.

I will never know what my dad and Lou talked about. But two
days later, their decision was made. Someone, probably Lou, phoned
Freeman with the news, which he recorded in his notes: "Mr. and
Mrs. Dully have apparently decided to have Howard operated on; I
suggested they come in for further discussions and not tell Howard
anything about it."

My uncle Orville told me many years later that my dad told him
that he "felt like God" when he signed the papers giving Freeman
permission to give me the lobotomy.

The following week my father and stepmother visited
Freeman together for the first time, to discuss my lobotomy.

Mr. Dully came in with Mrs. Dully today to talk over Howard's
forthcoming operation as they are convinced something will
have to be done. Mrs. Robinson [this was Lou's sister] called up
shortly before and stressed the need of tender, loving care after
Howard was operated on, and I assured her that everything
would be done.

Mr. and Mrs. Dully said that Howard was rather disap-
pointed that he wasn't going to come in for a further interview
today but I suggested it be postponed for a week, and that I will
tell him he has to go to the hospital for a series of examinations
and spend the night there. I called Doctors Hospital to make
arrangements . . .

On December 14, I visited Freeman with my father and Lou.
We saw Freeman separately. I must have waited while they saw him
first. According to Freeman's notes, the family had some second
thoughts about what was about to happen.

Howard is behaving much better this past week or two, and really pleasant at times, so that the family has had doubts about the desirability of his going through with the operation. These doubts were enhanced by the attitude of the minister and also of an aunt, but one of Mr. Dully's cousins knew somebody who'd been operated on and she is much better, so having no real encouragement from other sources, Mr. Dully has decided to go through with the operation.

It was like the train had already left the station, and everyone knew about it but me. I was the only person on the train, and I was the only one who didn't know where it was going. It was agreed that no one would tell me about the operation.

Then Freeman had me come in for one final chat.

I asked Howard about his recollections of his own mother and he was able to give me a few rather objective details but he didn't go into any discussion of his attitude toward her and his desperation at losing her. He says that he recently had the experience of hearing somebody in his room rather angrily talking at him; he turned on the light and there was nobody there. He doesn't remember the words but he was very alarmed. In regard to talking to himself he says he just talks to himself; he doesn't answer any spirit voices. He has a certain fascination with license plate numbers and also with words like "spring" that have a number of different meanings. I told him he was going into the hospital for some examinations; he was first afraid he might be hurt, but then glad that he'd be missing school.

That was Freeman's last entry before my lobotomy. I was going into the hospital for some examinations.

I liked the idea. I liked the attention. I'd get to miss school. I'd get fussed over in the hospital by a bunch of cute nurses in white uniforms. I'd get to lie in bed and watch TV. Plus I'd get to eat hospital food. I'd probably get to eat Jell-O, which we never had at home.

The hospital would be an adventure. I knew there was nothing wrong with me, so there was nothing to be afraid of. It couldn't be anything bad. If it was going to be something bad, they'd tell me—my dad, or Freeman, at least—right?

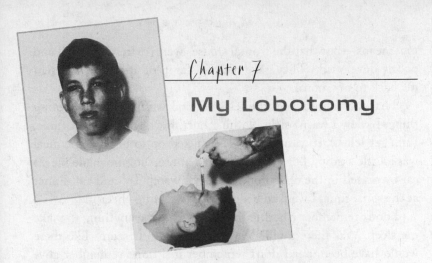

Chapter 7

My Lobotomy

Doctors General Hospital is a small private institution in San Jose. It looks more like a set of doctors' offices than a hospital. It's a long, low building, painted all white, with room for maybe fifty or sixty patients.

I was admitted as one of them on the afternoon of Thursday, December 15, 1960.

My dad drove me down there. Lou stayed home. I don't remember saying good-bye to her, or to George or Brian. I do remember having a sense of adventure, of playing hooky. I got to go to the hospital and they didn't. They had to go to school.

It was a sunny day, and my impressions of the hospital are all sunny ones. After we did the admitting paperwork, they put me in a bright, yellow room. My dad said good-bye without making any big deal out of it, and I was on my own.

I got undressed and put on the gown with the opening in back, which felt kind of ridiculous. Just like I'd expected, there were nurses clucking over me.

It was a private room, so I got to watch whatever I wanted on TV. But after a while I was interrupted by the nurses, who said the doctors had to do some tests. They took some blood. They listened to my heart. Then I went down to another room where they took some X-rays of my chest and then my head. The radiologist noted that my skull was normal, my pineal was not visualized—whatever *that* means—but that the frontal sinuses were "extremely small and poorly developed." They gave me the stamp of approval, and sent me back to my room.

That's it? Those were the tests? *Fine.* I wasn't worried about a thing. I knew I wasn't sick. Nothing hurt. Plus, when dinner came, I *did* get Jell-O. It wasn't all it was cracked up to be, and the meal was a little skimpy, but no one shouted at me. No one made me go eat by myself in the other room. I got to watch TV and eat dinner at the same time. I went to bed that night feeling cheerful.

I don't remember whether the nurses gave me anything to make me sleep. Was there a pill? Was there a shot? It seems like there would have been, but I don't remember it. I don't remember anything that happened next.

Freeman's admittance orders, written on the stationery bearing his 15 Main Street address in Los Altos, said this: "Please admit to Doctors Hospital Thurs. Dec. 15 at 3pm for transorbital lobotomy Dec. 16 at 1:30pm." His pre-op orders called for a complete blood count, measuring the "bleeding and clotting times," a urinalysis, an X-ray of my skull, and an electrocardiogram.

So far, so good. Then it says, "May be up and about until time for operation. Regular diet. If restless at night give him sodium amytal at 10:30." Sodium amytal is a barbiturate; it would certainly sedate me. That makes sense, too.

But Freeman had a warning for the nurses: "Avoid escape. The patient is full of tricks. Nurse not to leave him alone at any time. Is not to know why he is in the hospital except for examinations."

Escape? Why would I try to escape? Where would I go? I was a twelve-year-old kid in a hospital gown. My father and stepmother and doctor had all told me I was in the hospital for tests. I had no reason to believe they were lying to me. They were treating me like the Birdman of Alcatraz, but I was just a kid who had been looking forward to Jell-O.

I don't remember waking up the next morning. I don't remember being prepared for surgery. I don't remember seeing Freeman. I don't remember anything of that morning. That whole Friday disappeared.

Then it was over.

I remember waking up the next day, which would have been Saturday. I felt bad. My head hurt. I had a fever. They kept taking blood, and giving me shots. I thought something had gone wrong. What happened with the tests?

Freeman's notes tell the story: "Howard entered Doctors Hospital on the 15th and yesterday I performed transorbital lobotomy. The only thing that seemed to bother Howard was the needles he'd received on several occasions."

Freeman was assisted in the operating room by Dr. Robert Lichtenstein. His notes on the procedure sounded almost like a carpentry project:

> *I introduced the orbitoclasts [the name Freeman had given to his personally designed lobotomy knives] under the eyelids 3 cm from the midline, aimed them parallel with the nose and drove them to a depth of 5 cm. I pulled the handles laterally, returned them halfway and drove them 2 cm deeper. Here I touched the handles over the nose, separated them 45 degrees and elevated them 50 degrees, bringing them parallel for photography before removal.*

In other words, he poked these knitting needles into my skull, through my eye sockets, and then swirled them around until he felt he had scrambled things up enough. Then he took a picture of me with the needles in, and that was that.

To get me properly sedated, Freeman had administered a few jolts of electroshock. I don't know how much was typical, but I got some extra.

"Howard came around quickly after the first shock," Freeman wrote. "I eventually gave him four, after which he was quite slow in recovering. I think it was one more than necessary."

After the procedure, Freeman wrote that there was "an escape of a small amount of blood-stained fluid" from each eye socket. I did not get much swelling, he said. "However, he did have a considerable amount of vomiting during the night and I prescribed Dramamine 50 mg for its control. He'd been incontinent once during the night. He resisted efforts to get his eyes open and complained about the needles that were being given him. His temperature, pulse and respiration were quite normal."

My brain wasn't. Freeman said that I didn't know where I was or what was going on. "When I saw him this morning, he recognized me but thought he was on Orange Street and that the day was Monday instead of Saturday. He did not know that anything particular had happened to him."

Well, I knew *something* had happened, because I felt terrible. I may have picked up some kind of infection. Freeman's next set of notes, written the following Wednesday, read, "Howard had a rough time of it over the weekend. His temperature went up to 102.4 degrees, his neck was stiff; he had severe headache and was quite sluggish. I did a spinal puncture which showed some 4,000 white cells and 90,000 red cells, but the culture was sterile. During the waiting period for the culture I had given him about five or six doses of penicillin, 1 million units each, and his temperature promptly came down and stayed down."

Freeman was sort of famous, or infamous, for that "spinal puncture." Years before he had developed something he called the "jiffy spinal tap." Though he was accused from the beginning of risking his patients' lives using it, he liked this procedure for the same reason he liked the transorbital lobotomy: It was quick, and cheap, and didn't require an operating room or an assisting physician. With his "jiffy" procedure, Freeman simply had his patient sit in a chair turned around backward, with his head bent forward and his chin resting on his hands. Freeman then punctured the spinal column with a needle and entered the spinal canal at the base of the skull, between the first vertebra and the skull itself. As one medical writer said in his study of lobotomy, "A slight error (in this procedure) can produce a life-threatening injury."

The spinal tap, the infection, and the excess electroshock had left me pretty weak. Freeman's notes on my discharge read, "He was a bit wobbly on his feet when he was discharged from the hospital but was eating well, sleeping well and had no complaint of headache; his neck had loosened up and he seemed quite mild."

From reading Freeman's other notes I know the procedure didn't last more than ten minutes. There are no medical records available about my stay in Doctors General Hospital, so there is nothing but Freeman's notes to explain the fever and headaches and nausea.

But I do have a receipt, a "Physician's Service Report," from Blue Cross Hospital Service of California. It says that I was admitted on December 15 to be treated for "schizophrenia, mixed" and discharged on December 21. Under the heading of "Medical Treatment Rendered," the paper says, "Transorbital lobotomy. A sharp instrument was thrust through the orbital roof on both sides and moved so as to sever the brain pathways in the frontal lobes."

The charge for the hospital stay was two hundred dollars.

I don't remember coming home from the hospital. Neither does Brian. He wasn't there. Lou had him sent away, maybe because he'd broken down in Dr. Lopes's office. He remembers being gone about a week. When he came back, I was already home. My parents brought him upstairs, where I was tucked into my bed.

"You were sitting up in the bed, with two black eyes," Brian said later. "You looked listless. And sad. Like a zombie. It's not a nice word to use, but it's the only word to use. You were zoned out and staring. I was in shock. And sad. It was just terribly sad."

Brian couldn't remember what explanation Lou or my dad gave him for my condition. He thought they told him I was going to have an operation, something that would make me less angry.

George, being older, was given a little more information. He had been told I was going in for an operation. Lou said they were going to separate the two halves of my brain so I would stop being so "violent." George was frightened by that. He didn't think I was so violent. I was no more violent than he was. He knew that Lou got mad at me a lot, and that sometimes I got punished for things I didn't do. He was afraid they were going to hurt me. He may have been afraid they might hurt him, too. When he saw my black eyes and what shape I was in, George was scared.

I might have been a zombie for a while, but I was not a vegetable. The fight had not gone out of me. Freeman's next notes, on December 24, are short: "Howard is a bit of a handful, screaming at Mrs. Black and throwing a pillow at her, striking her on the arm and so on when she became too attentive; other than this, he is quite indolent, but he eats and sleeps and smiles well."

I don't have any memory at all of the days and weeks that followed. It was as if a fog had settled on me. I don't remember being in pain. I don't remember being unhappy. I don't remember convalescing. Was I in bed? Were people taking care of me? Other than the reference to me hitting Orville's wife, Evelyn, with a pillow, there's no information available to help me remember.

This was the beginning of what Freeman referred to as "the echo period." He said in his notes and his writings that this was a delicate time, following the surgery, when patients must be treated with great care. He had told my father and stepmother that they had to be very gentle with me during this period. I wasn't supposed to be put under stress. I wasn't supposed to be yelled at. I was supposed to be babied.

But on January 4, I was back in Freeman's offices. It was time for him to tell me what had happened. His entry for that day said: "I told Howard what I'd done to him today and he took it without a quiver."

So now I knew. But, did I? It was only a couple of weeks since the operation. And I was barely twelve years old. How conscious was I? How much could I understand? I wish I remembered.

Freeman's notes continued: "Also I discussed his activities in front of his parents, much to their concern since Howard has always shown such intolerance to open discussion of his activities. He's smiling a bit better and he says he doesn't hate George or his step-mother as much as he used to; he can hardly understand it himself since they still bore in on him."

All the way back to the first lobotomies, when Freeman was still drilling holes in people's skulls to do the surgery, he reported that his patients became almost immediately uninterested in the problems that used to make them crazy. The problems were still there but they no longer cared about them. One of Freeman's first patients became hysterical when they told her, the day before the surgery, that they'd have to shave part of her head to do the operation. She had to be restrained and sedated. A few days later, she was laughing about her bald spots, and thought it was silly that she'd ever been worried about them.

I seemed to have a similar reaction. I was not troubled by anything, Freeman wrote. I seemed almost happy, he said. "He says he doesn't have time to do much hating because he spends practically all day in front of the television. He still grumbles a bit if a different station is turned on. On the occasion of the Rose Bowl game he thoughtlessly went between his father and the television screen and jumped when his father yelled at him and apologized. He seems more easy to get close to and when his father puts him to bed and gives him a little rubbing or a gentle pat he seems to accept this."

Freeman went on to say that I was getting along well with Orville but not with Evelyn, so I guess I was back to spending Sundays with them. He also noted that I still teased the dog, and sometimes even teased Kirk. Freeman called these "hangovers" from my "previous activities," and said he advised Lou to "do a little yelling on her own." He added that my dad wanted a tutor to come in for a few hours a day. Freeman said he saw no problem with this. He concluded by saying, "Howard looks quite relaxed; he sleeps well, eats well and no longer gives the spine-chilling looks at his stepmother."

Freeman may have been trying to convince himself that I was all better. He was going to have a hard job convincing his medical colleagues.

A week after that visit with me and my parents, Freeman came to the house to pick me up in his car. We were going to drive up to San Francisco, for a presentation at the Langley Porter Clinic.

Along the way, we picked up two other young lobotomy patients. I didn't know them, and hadn't met them before. Richard was about sixteen, Ann was about fourteen.

I was excited to be going somewhere. Freeman talked the whole way up, not about anything in particular. I got the idea that we were going to some kind of a meeting to talk to people about our operations. Since I always liked it when Freeman wanted me to talk about me, I was happy to go along.

Freeman recorded in his notes that I seemed interested only in road signs, the length of the drive, the populations of the cities we were driving through, and the map of our journey.

When we got there, it wasn't what I expected. It was a big auditorium, and it was full. The seats were raised, angling away from the stage, almost like an operating theater, so that everyone was looking down on us. There were a lot of people there.

We sat on chairs onstage with Freeman off to the side, standing behind a podium with his notes. He talked a little bit about what he had done to us. He asked each of us a few questions. He recorded that I answered "in quite a low voice, and didn't have very much to say."

Neither did Richard. Maybe he got freaked out by all the people, or the lights. He wasn't able to answer the questions Freeman asked him. Freeman got frustrated, and pushed him to try harder. Richard said, "I'm doing the best I can." Freeman pushed him to try again.

Someone in the audience shouted something. Freeman explained that we had all had our surgeries quite recently, and besides, we were only children. Someone asked him how old I was—remember, I was a big kid. When Freeman said I had just turned twelve, the doctors were shocked. Only twelve? It was outrageous. The doctors started shouting and yelling. Freeman shouted back. Soon the whole place seemed out of control.

I thought we had done something bad. Other than Lou and my dad, I wasn't used to seeing adults lose their temper.

And Freeman really lost his. He had brought a box with him, and he suddenly pulled it out and dumped it onto the stage. It was filled with cards—Christmas cards, birthday cards, greeting cards of all kinds—hundreds of them.

"These are from my patients!" Freeman shouted. "How many Christmas cards do you get from *your* patients?"

He was booed off the stage. We got into the car and drove home.

Freeman later wrote his autobiography—it was never published, but I was able to see some of the pages from it—and he included his memories of the episode at Langley Porter. He said the audience response surprised him.

"I thought I had made a favorable impression," Freeman wrote. "Such was far from the case. The staff and residents at the institute are steeped in the Freudian tradition, and I was met with a barrage of criticism. Even when I pointed out that these youngsters were adjusting reasonably well at home and some of them even attending school, the specter of damaged brains prevailed. I had with me a box of Christmas cards, over 500 of them, and dumped them on the table. I had lost my temper. . . ."

His notes for the day added that when he got me back home, he presented me with a pocket knife. I told him that I already had two, but that my stepmother had hidden one and my uncle had taken away the other.

"I asked Mrs. Dully about the desirability of him having a knife and she said that he'd jabbed the furniture with a pencil and made deep scratches in it. I told her to see that Howard used it only outside, and to let me know if anything disagreeable happened."

For the next couple of months the "fog" continued, and so did my stepmother's irritation with me. I'm not sure why. Even Freeman's notes seem to suggest I was easier to get along with.

"Mrs. Dully came in with Howard and he seems to have grown another inch," Freeman wrote on February 4, 1961.

He sits quietly, grinning most of the time and offering nothing. Once in a while, when asked a direct question, he answers, "I don't know." Something happened to his bicycle tire so he hasn't been able to ride that, and he mostly stays around the house, goes outdoors and plays basketball and entertains himself pretty well while the other boys are away, and doesn't get into as many fights with them. It is a little hard on Mrs. Dully, who has to be there all the time, but Mr. Dully seems to be able to shrug it off pretty well. Mrs. Dully is not an affectionate sort of person nor demonstrative, and Howard certainly isn't, but it will take a while to get a greater degree of acceptance on the part of his family for Howard. At the present time they are inclined to call him lazy, stupid, dummy and so on, but Howard seems rather serene through all this and doesn't seem to be upset by such things. He doesn't go off and sulk and brood over things. He's sleeping well and eating well, although his table manners are deplorable.

My memory was still shaky, and I don't remember very much from this period. I know my bicycle was important to me, because my bicycle meant my freedom. I must have gotten it fixed, and I was allowed to ride almost anywhere I wanted. I could take the bike and ride up into the foothills, and be gone half a day without anyone asking where I'd been. When I was gone, no one was around to tell me what to do, or call me lazy, stupid, dummy, or anything else. I remember taking lots of long, long rides.

Whether Lou appreciated these breaks as much as I did, I don't know. But now that I'd had the surgery, she seemed even more frustrated by her inability to make me the boy she wanted me to be.

"Howard is getting his stepmother down," Freeman wrote a month later.

But I notice a great change for the better. He's much more open; he writes and draws better, is more responsive, smiles and, according to his father, is really less trouble in the home than he used to be. Nevertheless, Mrs. Dully says she has to spend all her

*time keeping Howard separated from the other boys since his be-
havior with them is difficult in the extreme. There is a plan to
find a foster home for Howard; it may be with the Blacks since
Mr. Black is so stable although his wife is an unsettling person.
I believe Howard will be able to stand this provided he has a
room to himself and this may be the fly in the ointment. I called
Family Service in Palo Alto and they referred me to the Welfare Department in San Jose. . . . Evidently Mrs. Dully needs
a rest.*

My memory began to return to me that spring. It's 1961. I remember the music on the radio. I can hear Ben E. King singing
"Stand by Me," and Dion singing "The Wanderer" and "Run-
around Sue." There was Del Shannon's haunting "Runaway," and
the sad "Daddy's Home" by Shep and the Limelites. It was a great
time for music. Ray Charles did "Hit the Road Jack" and Ricky
Nelson, one of my favorite singers, did "Hello Mary Lou."

But the pressure at home continued. By April, Lou had found a
way to throw me out of the house.

She found a home for me with a family named McGraw. Mrs.
McGraw was an old lady with red hair and glasses who ran a sort of
home away from home for kids. She lived on Sunshine Drive in
Los Altos, only about ten blocks or so from my house. Her husband
was a chubby, quiet guy who worked for the post office.

I liked it there. The McGraws had two sons named Danny and
Tommy. They were about eleven and twelve, and we had fun to-
gether. They went to school. I didn't. A "home teacher" named
Mrs. Van Horn came in to tutor me for a couple of hours a day.
There were also these two little girls, preschool age, who came to
Mrs. McGraw's for day care.

It seemed like my family liked the arrangement, too. Dr.
Freeman ran into my dad one afternoon in May at Whitecliff
Market, probably when my dad was bagging his groceries. Freeman
made a note that "the family has had five weeks of peace."

They must have liked that peace. I stayed with Mrs. McGraw for several months. I would have stayed longer, but there were several problems with the arrangement.

First was the financial problem. It cost quite a bit to keep a kid like me in a private home. (I learned later that Mrs. McGraw charged six dollars a day for my care.) My parents didn't want to spend the money, or couldn't afford to spend the money.

Second was the question of my dad's pride. It disturbed him that I wasn't a behavioral problem when I lived at Mrs. McGraw's, or when I was with Uncle Orville. He didn't want to admit that someone else might be able to raise his child better than he could. He was hardheaded, and a do-it-yourself kind of person. He couldn't accept that another person or another family could do the job better than him.

So he and Lou tried to get me placed in a state mental hospital.

At their request, Freeman wrote a letter to the superintendent of Napa State Hospital in March, asking him to take me on as a resident patient. "Howard Dully is now 12 years old and a schizophrenic since the age of four," the letter said. "His behavior was improved for a month or so after I performed transorbital lobotomy on him December 16, 1960, but he is going through the echo period and his step-mother cannot endure his behavior. There seems to be no foster home available."

Napa was willing to play along. The superintendent wrote back to Freeman, and urged him to have my family bring me in for an evaluation later that month.

I don't remember going in for the examination, but I must have. The doctors reported back a while later that I was not qualified for residence at the Napa mental institution.

"We did not find him psychotic," the superintendent wrote to Freeman. "He is not suitable for hospitalization."

Freeman suggested to my family that they try to get the government to foot the bill for my stay at Mrs. McGraw's. The superintendent at Napa had another idea: He wrote to Santa Clara County to ask whether I might be made a ward of the court, then adopted by Mrs. McGraw, so that I could stay on there without it costing my parents anything. The county would pay Mrs. McGraw for my care.

The plan took months to organize. There were letters back and forth. Napa State Hospital's superintendent sent letters repeating his opinion that I was not psychotic, but suggesting to the county that Mrs. McGraw would adopt me or become my official foster parent if my parents would agree to make me a ward of the state.

That didn't happen, but a suitable alternative emerged. I was declared a "dependent child." This is the category usually reserved for kids who are abused, malnourished, or otherwise not safe living at home. In my case, it seems like it was a question of money. My family could not have me at home, but they couldn't afford to pay Mrs. McGraw's rate, so the county declared me a dependent child, and that qualified me, or my family, for assistance. On May 24, 1961, my parents agreed to pay the county of Santa Clara $100 a month for my care. Since Mrs. McGraw was costing them at least $180 a month, that was a healthy reduction. There was more coming. A few months later, while I was still with Mrs. McGraw, the county agreed that the $100 a month was a hardship, and reduced it to $70 a month.

That took care of the financial side. But there was a third problem. Mrs. McGraw was very spiritual. My father said she was a "religious nut." She had me going to church all the time, and Sunday school. I didn't mind too much. I liked being away from Lou, and not being in trouble all the time, and it wasn't hard to stay out of trouble with Mrs. McGraw. If a little church time was part of the bargain, that was okay with me.

Not with my dad. He was complaining to Lou, and she was complaining to Freeman, that Mrs. McGraw was unstable and that she was making it difficult for him to see me. In handwritten notes following visits from Lou that spring, Freeman wrote about a conversation Lou had with my father:

*The woman with whom [Howard] has been living is, they feel,
a religious "nut," currently a Baptist, but changing churches whenever her own needs are unsatisfied. Both she and Howard's home
teacher have convinced each other that there's no reason in the
world why Howard can't return to school. Mr. Dully says it's getting to be that the woman where Howard is almost demands a
court authorization to let him see Howard.*

The religious stuff troubled my dad a lot. Even though he had
grown up with his mother's Christian Science, he was very opposed
to any other kind of organized religion. Since I was little I could remember him bad-mouthing church people, talking down Catholics
and Protestants alike. Forty years later, he would still get huffy
when his brother talked to him about going to church. So he certainly wasn't going to stand by while some woman enrolled his son
in a church school, and he wasn't going to have any Mrs. McGraw
tell him when he could or couldn't see his son.

So he decided he wanted me to come back home.

My condition seemed to be improving. Freeman saw me in
June. He wrote:

*Howard shows a most gratifying change in his attitude. He's re-
laxed and smiling, quite talkative, even to the point where I
have to interrupt him when he goes off into long discourses of
Danny and Tommy . . .*

*   There is a lively, graceful inflection of Howard's talk and the
lines of strain are gone. He's certainly doing wonders under the
care of Mrs. McGraw even tho' he rather objects to the dashing
here, dashing there, and insistence on church, when he would like
to be doing other things. He seems to get along well with the other
boys but rather misses George. Mr. Dully would like to have him
back in the family again but knows better than to try this at the
present time because Mrs. Dully is not yet accustomed to the idea.
Meantime Mr. Dully tells me that his former mother-in-law
(Howard's grandmother) is stirring things up in Oakland and*

trying to get the Alameda Co. Medical Society interested in my nefarious doings.

This was my grandmother Daisy Patrician, my mom's mother. She was still living in Oakland. She had not been around much, as far as I know, but when she got word of what had happened to me she got mad. I guess she objected to the idea of someone giving a lobotomy to a twelve-year-old kid—at least if the kid was her grandson.

Daisy started writing letters. She wrote to my father and accused him of concealing my whereabouts from her, and concealing the facts about my surgery. He was conducting "a conspiracy of culpable malpractice and avoidance of parental duty." She wrote to hospital administrators, saying, "Howard has been removed from school and no longer manifests the natural personality his relatives had known as the human being, Howard Dully, but rather a strange disinterested being, foreign to his youthful age." She demanded to know who allowed the surgery to go forward. "Who can assume or give moral authority and take responsibility for such an act?"

When she wrote to Freeman, he agreed to see her—but advised her that he would charge twenty-five dollars for the consultation. Daisy was outraged. She wrote to the Santa Clara County Medical Society, demanding to see Freeman's credentials and threatening to have them taken away.

I don't know whether my dad and Lou hired a lawyer, but Freeman started consulting with one immediately. It quickly became clear that my dad would back Freeman, who assured the lawyer that my grandmother had been "a disturbing influence" throughout his marriage to June, and that she had not been consulted on the question of my lobotomy, and that he was willing to state on the record that "everything was done for the welfare of the lad." The correspondence between Freeman and the lawyer concludes, "Mr. Dully says that he is not concerned."

There was at least one face-to-face meeting in the house between Daisy and my dad. My little brother Brian witnessed it—or at least he witnessed it with his *ears*. He said there was an argument like nothing he'd ever heard in his life. My dad and Daisy screamed and yelled. My dad was brutal. He told Daisy he knew about her son Gordon's earlier plan to take me and Brian away from him. He told Daisy he knew Gordon was a homosexual. He called Gordon some names. Daisy fought back, but she was no match. Brian said my father screamed her right out of the house.

Freeman's notes from later that month support Brian's memory of that episode. Lou visited with him around that time. Freeman wrote, "Mrs. Dully said that when her husband's former mother-in-law came down and started reading the riot act about Howard he gave her what-for and shouted louder than she did, so they haven't heard a peep out of her since."

It didn't stay that quiet. Freeman was contacted by his insurance company, which held the policy on his malpractice insurance. They had been contacted by the Alameda-Contra Costa County Medical Association, which had received a complaint and claim of malpractice from a Mrs. Daisy Patrician. The insurance adjuster wanted to meet with Freeman *immediately*.

I don't know how or when the situation was resolved. Daisy kept at it for at least the next four years. When she became exasperated, her son Gordon started writing letters, too, demanding information and threatening legal action.

It must have been a nightmare for my father. Daisy was threatening a lawsuit. Mrs. McGraw wanted me to stay with her, but that was still costing my family seventy dollars a month, which they couldn't afford to spend. Worse, Mrs. McGraw had stated her intention to start me in a church school come September. She was not willing to keep me on otherwise.

In August, I was still living with Mrs. McGraw, but my dad had made his mind up that once the school year started, I had to come back home and start attending Covington again.

Lou didn't like this one bit. But what could she do? She had tried everything in her power to get rid of me. She had said everything she could say against me. So she used the only weapon she had left: She threatened to move out if I moved back in.

"Mrs. Dully came in today and laid it on the line," Freeman wrote in August, 1961. "She says the past four months when Howard has been out of the family has been a period of mutual relaxation and friendly feeling. It seems that Mr. Dully has more or less made up his mind that when September arrives and the school year begins, Howard is going to leave Mrs. McGraw and come back home. Mrs. Dully finds it rather unacceptable and wonders whether she would be better out of the way . . ."

As the month wore on, so did her resolve against having me home. My dad was insisting on having me back in the house. Lou was dead-set against it.

"Mrs. Dully has let her husband know that she won't tolerate Howard in the house, and bristles at the very thought of it," Freeman wrote after another visit.

> *Mr. Dully says that Howard has changed radically in the past few months and that he is no longer surly, preoccupied and teasing, nagging, destructive or critical, but sort of friendly in superficial ways so that his father has a stronger liking for him than ever and has never been called upon to punish the boy for infractions of discipline.*
>
> *The word . . . from Mrs. McGraw is that Howard is getting along well with the two boys, but because of the religious fanaticism Mr. Dully is not able to get any exact description. However, Howard seems quite unaware of any tendency to get into arguments or fights. Howard seems to have no particular depth of feeling about anything. He is rather indifferent to looking forward to school.*

In his notes, Freeman said there had been conversation about a counterproposal: Maybe my dad's uncle Frank, who was now living in Centralia, Washington, would be willing to take me on. Frank and his wife had already taken over the care of my little brother Bruce, who was now eight years old. Uncle Frank had been trying to get Bruce accepted at an institution of some kind. Maybe I could move up there once Bruce had been placed in a home.

My dad told Freeman why my uncle wanted me to move up there with him.

"He is fire chief and has a good deal of time on his hands which he devotes to the care of Howard's younger brother," Freeman wrote in August. "But he wants a boy that can grow up and fish and hunt and be outdoors with him."

My dad and Lou were going off on a vacation shortly, a driving tour with George, Brian, and Kirk. They were going to drive as far as Washington State, and my dad was going to have a talk with Uncle Frank. I wasn't invited. I didn't go. I stayed with either Mrs. McGraw or my uncle Gene.

The driving trip came and went. The plan to move me failed. My dad reported to Freeman after he got back that his uncle Frank had decided not to invite me to live with him in Washington.

Freeman continued to do what he could to help keep me out of the house. He wrote a letter to my parents in September 1961 that was obviously meant to be read by someone else. It seemed like my dad and Lou were going to submit the letter to some institution or foster home, to show what a good boy I was.

Freeman's letter said:

> I have had the chance on a number of occasions to watch the development of your son Howard from a surly, antagonistic, suspicious, teasing, lying, and generally disagreeable person into a smiling, unselfconscious, alert and cooperative youngster who has become progressively more integrated with others about him. . . . I attribute [this] to the operation I performed on him eight months ago.
>
> Unfortunately the home situation has been so colored by the reactions to Howard's presence in the past that I recommend strongly against his going back into your home. I foresee, if that

occurs, a relapse into previous irritating and even explosive
events which could easily set Howard back . . .

I don't know who got the letter, or why I wasn't put into a foster home. But in the end it was decided that I would move in with my uncle Gene and his family, across town in the city of San Jose, where I would start school, in the seventh grade again, at Herbert Hoover Junior High.

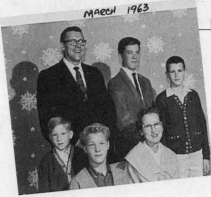

MARCH 1963

Chapter 8

Big Enough
and
Ugly Enough

Uncle Gene was my dad's older brother, the oldest of the three Dully boys. He was a good man. He looked like an Italian—dark and smooth. He liked kids. He worked with the YMCA, and he spent a lot of time with his son Frank, who was about fourteen, and his two stepsons, Dennis and Pinky, who were about thirteen and eleven. Uncle Gene was not a man who would belittle you, like my dad. He showed kids some respect.

I don't know what he told his sons about what happened to me, or about why I was moving in, and I don't know what he told the people at Herbert Hoover. It was never discussed with me. I was never teased about it. No one ever asked me what it felt like to have a lobotomy. It never came up. I was treated just like any other kid.

Like my dad, Gene was a schoolteacher. He taught middle school in Los Altos. (Kenny, my dad's other brother, worked at IBM.) But he wasn't sick of kids or tired all the time when he got home, or working after school every day, like my dad. He still had time for Little League and stuff like that.

I didn't get into trouble at Uncle Gene's. I remember being punished once. I think I was caught in a lie, and I got spanked. But that was it. I went from being in trouble all the time, and being punished all the time, to doing all right at Mrs. McGraw's, then doing all right with Uncle Gene.

That's not to say there wasn't some trouble here and there. According to Freeman, I was having difficulties at school.

"Howard is now living with his father's older brother, Mr. and Mrs. Eugene Dully," he wrote in January 1962.

I talked with them for about an hour on the subject of Howard, who is in difficulties with school, not so much because he doesn't know enough—he is doing ninth grade reading and eighth grade arithmetic—but he forgets his books and his pencils and has failed in all his subjects except one. He has a sympathetic teacher and doesn't show any of his hostility, but his peculiarities of behavior have gotten him many visits to the principal and have tended to exhaust his teachers. He uses his lunch money to buy candy for the boys, he borrowed a bicycle without permission, he is clumsy, he doesn't join in games, he has poor posture, yet he is interested in girls and sometimes dances to the radio or TV. He is not inclined to stay too much to himself . . .

Howard seems to want a lot of attention, and when his father comes to see him, or take him out, he is quite affectionate. Howard is careless about the way he looks, he goes to school sometimes in his play clothes. He doesn't seem to try to learn, he is not disobedient or defiant, but he does need a paddling once in a while. Howard is really a non-conformist. The Dullys are hopeful that Howard will improve sufficiently so that with the reward of going home again held before him he will behave better. I asked them to bring Howard to see me.

They did, a week later.

Howard is taller every time I see him. He seems to be doing his school work all right, but he gets marked down in deportment so that there is only one class in which he excels. He has a sort of off-hand way of discussing his activities, but whether it is talking in class or slipping notes or shooting darts he must have a disquieting effect on the class. His athletic activities are also hampered by lack of skill and poise. He doesn't draw well, and is not interested in music. He says he gets along well enough with his cousins, but Mrs. Gene Dully is almost at her wits' end. Apparently Howard doesn't realize what a problem he is in his foster home. His father comes to see him every Tuesday, but he doesn't stay long and apparently isn't interested in the boy. Howard wants to go to his own home, but is certainly not ready for it.

Gene and his wife, Christine, lived in a little three-bedroom stucco house on a quiet street in San Jose just a few blocks from the junior high school, which was a big two-story Spanish-style building. It was an older school, not like the little bungalow-style school I had been going to, but big and stately. It felt like a real school, for grown-up kids.

Some of them were doing grown-up things. Even though it was just the seventh grade, there were kids "going steady." By the eighth grade they were "getting pinned," which meant they were exchanging these things known as "virgin pins." I never knew exactly what that meant, but the virgin pin was a circular gold pin that you'd wear on your jacket or sweater. It meant "I'm spoken for."

My cousin Frank got pinned. He came home and sat down at the dinner table wearing it. Uncle Gene came unglued. He said, "What the hell is that thing?" Frank explained what it was, and told him that all the kids at Herbert Hoover were exchanging virgin pins—that it was completely normal.

Uncle Gene didn't buy that. He was disgusted. He said, "And I suppose if they all started walking around with their peckers out, you'd do that, too? Take it off!"

I didn't get pinned, and I didn't have a girlfriend. But I was starting to have some thoughts in that direction.

It was while I was living at Uncle Gene's that I had my first sexual "accident." I was lying in bed, sort of fooling around and . . . Oh, boy.

At first I didn't know what I had done. But I knew it felt good. I didn't want to ask anybody what it meant. I was afraid they'd tell me to stop.

I'm not sure what I was thinking about at the time. It might have been one of my teachers. Her name was Mrs. Goldner, or maybe *Miss* Goldner. I had a big crush on her. She was tall and slender, and she reminded me of my mom. She dressed like my mom—not like Lou—in nice clothes. She had pretty hair, not dark like my mom's, but light-colored.

I fantasized a lot about what it would be like to be with her. I don't know if she was married or not. I didn't try to find out. I knew it was just a fantasy. It's not like I told her about it, or asked her out. I never said anything to her about it, or gave her any indication of how I felt, or told anyone else about it. I just imagined what it would be like to be with her.

Around girls my own age I was shy. Too shy. We had some dances at Herbert Hoover, and I'd go with Frank. But I didn't do anything. I didn't approach any of the girls. I didn't know what to say to them. Either they approached me or it didn't happen.

I had this theory. I figured *they* knew already whether they wanted to dance with me. So all they had to do was come up and tell me what they decided—yes or no. If it was no, they wouldn't come up at all. If it was yes, they would. So, I just stood there.

You don't get a lot of dates that way. You don't meet a lot of girls. Maybe that's why Frank got pinned and I didn't.

But I did get a kiss. While I was living at Uncle Gene's, I had my first real encounter with a girl. And I liked it.

I had a friend from school named Steve. One Saturday he invited me to come to the movies. He had this girl he was interested in, and she had a friend, so when he invited her to the movies he needed someone to be with the friend. I agreed to go.

It was awkward. I didn't know what to do. I didn't even know the girl's name. But somehow we wound up necking in the movie theater—right there in the Town Theater in downtown San Jose. I don't remember what the movie was, but I remember it was sort of crowded. It was crowded enough, anyway, that the girl was too shy to keep kissing with everyone looking. So I took off my jacket and put it over our heads. Steve and his girl did the same thing. We were all shy, I guess.

It was during this period that I began to disappear from the family photos. Back through the years there were snapshots taken of us, at holiday time, in the mountains at Easter time, and for birthdays and other occasions. Once my dad married Lou, the casual snapshots disappeared and the formally arranged photographs began. My dad was working at Kodak, and he always had a camera and film in the house. He would take the pictures, but Lou would set them up. She usually had us line up by height, Bink at the far left and Brian at the far right, with me next to Bink and George next to Brian. In all of them, we look miserable. There's one of us standing in pajamas that Lou had hand-sewn for us, dated June 1956. We look like we're lined up for a firing squad. There's another from a year later, April 1957, taken at Uncle Ross's cabin. We're arranged by height again, with the newly arrived baby Kirk being held by Bink—who looks just a little bit more unhappy than the rest of us. Another picture from three years later includes Lou standing between Bink and me. Everyone has a forced smile on except me. I have my eyes closed, a grimace on my face and my hands shoved into my pockets. The picture is dated March 1959.

Starting a year later, there are pictures from the house, from the cabin, and at holiday time, but I'm not there. A whole set from the summer of 1961—the summer after my lobotomy, the summer they went to Washington to visit my dad's uncle Frank, doesn't show me at all.

The next family photo I'm in is a holiday photo from several years later. George and Kirk are seated in front next to Lou, who's wearing a formal coat. Standing behind are Brian, wearing a cardigan, on the right, and my dad, wearing a suit and tie, on the left. I'm in the middle, wearing one of those hated corduroy jackets and a necktie. My dad has his characteristic family photo grin, and he looks like David Seville, the father figure from *Alvin and the Chipmunks*, or like the guy who played the dad on the TV show *Dennis the Menace*. The rest of us are almost completely expressionless. No one is smiling. George, Kirk, and Brian are looking at the camera steadily, like they don't trust it. I have a slightly demented smirk on my face, like I don't trust anybody.

I stayed at Uncle Gene's for the entire school year. I remember it being pretty good. The family was nice to me. My cousin Frank was okay. The kids at Herbert Hoover were okay. I know I missed George, and I know I missed being at home, but being at home meant being around Lou, and that was difficult for me.

Difficult for her, too, I guess. Freeman wrote in his notes that Lou saw me only two times during the six months I stayed with Mrs. McGraw. I don't think she saw me at all during the time I was at Uncle Gene's.

I continued to see Freeman from time to time, as did my uncle Gene and my Dad.

"Howard thinks he is doing pretty well in mathematics, mechanics and spelling," Freeman wrote in March 1962.

> *He is at ease and smiling, but his aunt says that he acts as if he were under a permanent tranquilizer. The boy has not learned how to tie his neckties and his uncle is rather resentful about this, nevertheless Howard grooms himself better and never gets mad. He is careless about books, pencils and so on, he has left jackets at school and also T-shirts in his locker, he is not doing his assignments [but] if Mr. Dully is sufficiently foresighted to remind him in time of what has to be done, he seems to get it done. He is getting along better with Mrs. Dully's boys and she did not suggest moving him out.*

That last part changed. By June, I was wearing out my welcome. Freeman wrote after meeting with my aunt, "She is of the opinion that she has done as much as she can for the boy. She says he is no more trouble than the other 3 boys that she has, but is different from them in that he is aloof."

My dad was reporting all kinds of progress. He ran into Freeman at the Whitecliff Market, where he was still working in the afternoons, and told him I was doing well. "Howard is giving up, one by one, his disagreeable traits," Freeman wrote. "He seems more considerate of others and while still careless with a good many faults yet to overcome, is improving all the time."

But there was new trouble at home. It had nothing to do with me. Lou had been sick.

After bumping into my father outside Whitecliff, Freeman wrote, "Later on I talked with Mrs. Dully, who has had a hysterectomy for cervical cancer and found that the home is always a quieter and pleasanter place after Howard has left, although he is so much better than he was a year ago that there is no comparison."

For Brian, this was the second time he was sent away from the house without really being told why. This time he was sent to live with Lou's mother, known as Granny, and the occasion was Lou's hysterectomy. Like me, he didn't know until he was an adult what the surgery was.

Much later I would wonder about Lou's headaches, her raging temper, and the other problems Freeman's notes said were "psychosomatic." Could these have been part of a larger medical problem? Could her difficulties with me have been part of that, too? My cousin Linda told me Lou was "a pharmacy in and of herself. She had a pill for everything. She was always on something." Could that have been the explanation for her treatment of me?

Despite my improvement, and Lou's recovery, I still wasn't welcome at home. It was still being talked about like it was a dangerous thing. But my father must have convinced Lou that it was necessary. When summer came and the school year at Hoover ended, I moved back home again. Freeman's notes from that August contain a new series of complaints against me from, of course, Lou. The notes indicate Freeman had a visit with both of us early that summer.

Howard has been home since the end of school and, according to Mrs. Dully, is much the same. He tyrannizes over the 2 little boys, Bryan and Kirk . . . Mrs. Dully says that Howard is liberal with the truth, that the two boys are frequently upset because Howard uses bad language, tells stories, messes up their rooms and seems to take some malicious pleasure in having them run to Mamma. Meantime, Mr. Dully has a job at Kodak; he is going to San Jose State and works on the garden over the weekends. Mrs. Dully thinks her husband is getting more upset with the passage of time and that she can't reach him anymore to sit down and talk over their problems. Mr. Dully is remarkably bad with Howard, criticizing him, yelling at him and seldom giving him a word of praise.

Howard says his mind is full of ideas but he hasn't set any of them down on paper, either in drawings or in stories. He is not athletic, and doesn't seem to pay much attention to girls. He is rather casual with his boy friends, spends a good deal of time in his room and keeps out of the way of his father. On the whole he is much the same.

I wasn't much the same. I was growing up. I was standing up to my father—Freeman reports that when we were doing yard work my father threw a pitchfork full of horse manure on me, so I threw a pitchforkful right back at him. I was using rougher language, maybe what I'd picked up hanging around the kids at Herbert Hoover.

Again they began discussing ways to get me out of the house. In August 1962, according to Freeman's notes, they started hunting for another foster home. They didn't find one. In January 1963, I was still at home, and Lou was still complaining.

"Mrs. Dully gave me the picture as she sees it with Howard," Freeman's notes read for January 30.

The boy is "just what he used to be." He contributes nothing, won't bathe, and the only difference she sees in him now is that he no longer plays with feces and is not vicious. He seems to take things and is getting worse and worse at school, so that the principal at Covington has suggested that, though he is in the 8th grade, he be shifted to the mental retardation group or altogether removed from school.

Mr. Dully does not take kindly to this and seems to believe that physical punishment will bring the boy around. [He] is quite punitive with the boy, saying he will whip him to death if necessary.

Mrs. Dully is fed up with the situation and is planning a separation unless Howard is removed from the family. She says her husband is losing his health and his sense of proportion and yet won't admit that there is any reason to eject Howard.

The tension between them must have been horrible. Lou wanted me out of the house and was threatening to leave the marriage if I didn't go. My dad still insisted he could get me into line with physical punishment. Freeman wrote that I spent a lot of time in my room trying to stay away from my father. I guess I would have. I remember those beatings.

I remember Lou exploding at me only once. She got angry at me over something. We were standing in the kitchen. All of a sudden she started screaming at me. "This is why we had you operated on! And you still won't behave! Go to your room!"

By February, the situation had become impossible for everyone. My dad was worn out. I was six feet tall now, and almost as big as my father, according to Freeman's files. Even though my father had "taken a stick" to me on several occasions, Freeman wrote, "the punishments have had no lasting effect, except to make Howard sore."

My size seems to have impressed everyone more than my age did. Freeman wrote in his notes about a meeting he had with my parents in which they all decided it was time for me to move into my own place.

With Howard and Mr. Dully present I said that Howard would have to leave his home, and that he was "big enough and ugly enough" to be established in a room of his own and with an al-lowance that he would have to get along on somehow, that he could no longer remain at home, would have to be rejected by the family in order to keep Mrs. Dully at home with the other boys. If Howard was unable to make the grade he would have to go to an institution.

The date on that entry is February 2, 1963. I might have been big enough and ugly enough in someone's mind. But I was just fourteen years old. I was having trouble in school. Freeman wrote that I got an A in spelling but a D in reading, and that I didn't seem to be able to apply myself. I contributed nothing in the home and didn't even bathe properly. But their solution was for me to move out and get a room of my own and start taking care of myself like a grown-up.

Freeman had left out or not been informed of some developments at home and at school. Things had taken a turn for the worse.

In September 1962 I had returned to Covington. There were a lot of teachers there I didn't like, and I *especially* didn't like Mr. Proctor, the civics teacher. So one day I designed a little weapon, and I shot him—using a rubber band and a paper clip. I ditched the weapon in the desk next to mine, an empty desk that no one used, so Proctor wouldn't know who did it.

He knew anyway. He didn't see me do it. He didn't find the weapon in my desk. There was no way he could know for sure who attacked him. But he knew. I guess I had a history with him. So he started asking for witnesses and taking statements. He conducted a mock trial right there in the classroom. No one would testify against me, but when it was over Proctor pronounced me guilty just the same. He marched me down to the principal's office and told him what I had done. I was suspended until the following Monday. I was told to get my things from the classroom and go home.

Well, I couldn't go home. I couldn't face Lou. She'd kill me for getting suspended. I knew my dad would find out soon enough about my being dismissed for the day. But that was no reason to go home early and get punished by Lou *now*.

I had this girlfriend at the time named Lori. We'd talk and hold hands. I felt safe with her. She lived near Hillview Elementary, which is not far from Covington. So I talked her into letting me have the key to her house. She lived alone with her mom, and her mom worked during the day, so the house would be empty. I could hang out there until school ended. Lori told me to just be very careful not to "disturb" anything. If her mom found out about me staying there during school time, she'd get into trouble.

I wasn't planning on disturbing anything, but I disturbed things plenty. I hung out for a while. I watched a little TV. I ate a snack and drank a soda. I got bored and started wandering around the house. There was nothing interesting about that. So I went to check out the backyard. The back door slammed shut, and I discovered I had locked myself out of the house.

There was a high fence around the whole yard—too high for me to climb over. I was tall, but I wasn't *that* tall. I couldn't hide in the backyard all day. Lori would be home soon. Her mother would be home soon. I had promised I wouldn't disturb anything, and now look what had happened.

I decided the best thing to do was get back into the house, straighten things up, and then leave through the front door. But I had locked myself out. The only way to get back in was to break a window. So I broke a window and let myself back in. But now there was a broken window. I put the key where Lori had told me to put it and I snuck out.

Did I think I wouldn't get caught? I don't know. I don't remember. But of course I got caught. Lori came home. Her mother came home. There was that broken window. Lori told her mother about letting me have the key. Lori's mom called my house and talked to Lou. My dad came home and Lou talked to him. All hell broke loose.

I don't know exactly what happened, but I didn't go back to school the following Monday. I couldn't. I was expelled. My father had spoken to the principal of the school that Friday afternoon. Somehow, their conversation got me thrown out of school. I was told not to return on Monday. I never went back.

It was the beginning of December. School would be out for winter break within two weeks. I figured, what the heck? I could get a couple of weeks off, and then in January I'd go back and try again. It didn't seem like that big a deal to me. What's a couple of weeks off from school? I spent the time on my own, away from the house, riding my bike up into the foothills, exploring, nobody telling me what to do. It was a good time.

It would be the last good time I had for a long time.

The next Freeman entry is February 6, 1963. It's a short note. It's ominous. It makes reference to Agnews—which could only mean the Agnews State Hospital. I knew about Agnews. It was the state hospital for the insane.

Freeman's note says, simply, "Mr. Dully is going to have Howard admitted to Agnews for a 10 day evaluation period. The school [Covington] definitely won't take him back and he cannot be managed at home. I told Mr. Dully I would be glad to supply the hospital with any information they wanted."

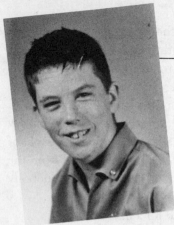

Chapter 9

Asylum

Agnews is a gigantic green park, not far from the railroad tracks in San Jose. Built in the 1880s, it is ninety acres of rolling lawns, huge cypress trees, and stately cream-colored Spanish buildings with red-tile roofs. These days, it's the world headquarters of the computer company Sun Microsystems.

Back then, it was called Agnews State Hospital, and was known as "the great asylum for the insane." It had housed mental patients for more than seventy years when I got there, surviving even the great San Francisco earthquake of 1906. Years later, I read newspaper stories about that. Several buildings collapsed, killing more than a hundred mental patients. When the shaking ended, the orderlies handcuffed the surviving patients to trees until the buildings were safe to enter again.

The day I arrived was a cold, bleak winter day, and I was wearing handcuffs.

I had already been locked up for a while, a veteran of Juvenile Hall, where my father and stepmother had taken me when they turned me over to the system.

After my father's last meeting with Freeman, he and Lou had started the paperwork to get the county of Santa Clara to make me a "ward of the court."

To do that, they had to make various declarations. They had to get my classification changed from 600, for "dependent child," to 601, for children who were "beyond control."

The 600 category was for kids who were in danger, or who needed to be removed from the home for their own safety. The 601 category was for kids who were causing too much trouble at home, or were at risk of becoming seriously delinquent. The 602 category was for kids who had already become delinquent, and who were hurting people or destroying things.

The State of California Superior Court document my parents signed said, "The father of said minor made an application for a Juvenile Court petition alleging that said minor is suspected of taking things from the home, refuses to obey reasonable and proper orders, is sarcastic and belligerent, and is beyond control at home and school . . ."

A companion document, the Application for Juvenile Court Petition, said,

Howard has been extremely belligerent toward his father and step-mother. He refuses to clean his room and come home immediately after school. He refuses to prepare, complete and turn in required school assignments and also causes classroom disturbances. The parents suspect him of stealing money and articles from his own home. On 2-4-63, the minor stole a gear shift knob from a parked automobile. The father, at this time, requests assistance of the Santa Clara County Juvenile Court in the control and possible placement of said minor.

The court agreed, and said it would spend two dollars a day to house me in Santa Clara County Juvenile Hall.

I was admitted there on February 14, 1963—Valentine's Day.

I knew all about Juvenile Hall—or "juvie," as the kids all called it. Any kid who's been in trouble knows about juvie. You hear about it the first time you get caught doing anything. "They're gonna send you to *juvie*, man!" I had heard that about a thousand times.

But I thought it was reserved for people who did something serious—robbed a gas station, or stole a car, or pulled a knife on someone. I didn't know you could get sent to Juvenile Hall, or made a ward of the court, for not doing your homework or having a stepmother who didn't like you.

My stepbrother Cleon had warned me about juvie. I think my dad made him talk to me, to try to scare me. He told me it was a terrible place. He gave me the idea that it was just a bunch of big guys hanging off the bars, waiting for a kid like me to show up. He made it sound like any kid who got sent there would be lucky not to be raped or have his throat cut the first day.

So I was scared.

I don't remember how I got there. But I remember arriving at this big, cold, white building, several stories high but almost completely windowless, near downtown San Jose. It looked like a prison.

They put me in a cell by myself, on the observation unit, and kept me there for three days. I couldn't see what kinds of people were there. I didn't know if they were going to be kids like me, or bigger kids, or adults hanging from the bars and drooling and waiting to hurt me.

There were no bars. The rooms were made of cinder blocks, with a cement floor. There was a bed and a nightstand. There was heat, but not much. The rooms were cold, and the whole environment felt cold. Metal and concrete. The door to the room was metal, with a window in it.

The only good thing was the food, and there was plenty of it. For the first few days, while I was under observation, they brought it to my cell on a tray. The tray had vegetables on it, but I didn't have to eat them. I got Jell-O! I remember thinking, *Hey, this isn't so bad.*

After three days I was moved into the regular environment, and placed in unit B-II, which housed about thirty kids. Some of the ones I met were there for real crimes—shoplifting and stealing. But most of the kids didn't say what they were there for, just like I didn't say. You didn't go around bragging about having a lobotomy, or about being thrown out of your house and made a ward of the court. And you didn't go around asking what the other kids were there for, either.

Each guy had his own cell. At mealtime, you'd walk down to the day hall and wait there in line. Then they'd march you down to the chow hall. Stand in line. Pick up a tray. They'd throw food on the tray. You'd sit at these long tables with the other guys from your section.

It was loud and aggressive, just like prison. The big boys would steal the little boys' dessert. There were fights. It was edgy.

At first it was very scary. I remember lying alone in my bed at night crying, wishing I wasn't there, wishing I was home. I missed my family.

I have a copy of a letter I wrote on February 21, 1963—a week after my arrival. The return address is Howard A. Dully, B-II, Cell 5. In the letter I talk about being questioned by a policeman. I wasn't accused of anything. But I was able to tell the policeman that I had been hanging out with a boy named John, who had been arrested for breaking into Covington High School and stealing things. I was going to try to sort it all out with my probation officer.

"John is now here and is sorry he did it," I wrote. "I am lucky I cut out when he told me what he was going to do. I am going to see my P.O. Thursday. I am not afraid now to tell the truth."

I don't remember any of this—the letter, the break-in, or even who John is. But the weird thing is the letter appears to be written directly to *Lou*. At the end it says, "Hope you are feeling well, and George, Brian, Kirk and Dad." The last line says, "I will draw some faces and enclose them in this letter, Love, Howard." Stapled to the letter is a set of four silly cartoon drawings of someone's face.

I guess I was reaching out. I was trying to make Lou love me.

We were kept busy during the day. We had to study, which I didn't like—math and English. I was bored. They'd tell me two plus two equals four. I got it. Then they'd tell me that two plus two equals four again. I got it! Or they'd tell me we were going to read a book, and they'd give me the book, and tell me to read it, and then they'd read it out loud. I hated that. You read the book, or you let *me* read the book. Not both!

They had a shop class, too, where they taught us to work with plastics. We made things like gear-shift knobs—like the ones I had stolen—for cars we would never own. It was great, even if it was only for an hour a day.

We had exercise time, too, out in the yard. There was basketball. I didn't do too much of that. I didn't like all that running around. I'm sociable when I'm around people I like and understand, and who don't scare me. At that time, in that place, I wasn't very sociable. I didn't make any friends.

But I did spend a lot of time talking to doctors, psychologists, and psychiatrists. They all wanted to know how I was feeling, what I was feeling, what I was thinking. Well, what do *you* think? I felt bad. I wanted out.

I think the authorities wanted me out, too. In March, the Santa Clara County Juvenile Probation Department's psychiatry division made its report on me. A psychiatrist named Dr. Shoor oversaw my evaluation. His assessment was a little different from Dr. Freeman's.

"The minor was brought into the Department by his father after making an unsuccessful attempt to get him into Napa State Hospital," Dr. Shoor's report says. "The father declared Howard as beyond control in that he is failing in school, constantly harasses his stepmother, terrifies his younger brother, suspects him of stealing, and stated that he could no longer keep him in his house. This move was triggered off when Dr. Freeman recommended to the father that Howard should have a room outside the home or he would destroy the family."

Dr. Shoor went on to review my situation. He noted that I had been very close to my mother, and that she had died when I was young. He said that before my operation "the parents (especially the stepmother) considered him intolerable to live with. It was the stepmother who initially took him to Dr. Freeman." The report mentions the transorbital lobotomy.

But the report doesn't end where most of the other reports had ended. Dr. Shoor wrote that I appeared to be "a seriously disturbed boy." He said, "The stepmother has always seen him as a problem and not nearly as good as her own sons. In the home at this time he is always looked on with skepticism and is never allowed to be alone with his younger brother. Neither parent feels they can trust him."

And so, Shoor concluded, "In the best interest of Howard, he should be removed from his home in that *his stepmother seems determined to destroy him.*"

Freeman attended the meeting where these findings were discussed, in the office of my juvenile probation officer, a Mr. W. Ellison. Dr. Shoor was there. So were my parents. Freeman's notes say that I had been at Juvenile Hall for three or four weeks. I learned later that Dr. Shoor hated Freeman, and hated the fact that he performed lobotomies on children, and wished it was in his power to stop him.

Freeman didn't mention that. He wrote in his notes for that day, "I agreed with Mrs. Dully that Howard was a danger in the home, but made no recommendation as regards the solution of the problem."

A solution was found, just the same. Because I was not a criminal, because I had not been charged with anything, the people at Juvenile Hall couldn't hold me. Because they'd determined I wasn't psychotic, Napa State Hospital wouldn't make room for me there. Because my dad wouldn't allow me to be adopted, I couldn't go live with the McGraws—the only family that seemed to want me.

So, somehow, the people in charge of my welfare decided I should be sent to Agnews, the great asylum for the insane.

I was driven from Juvenile Hall to Agnews by a probation officer. Before I got into the car, he handcuffed me—for my "protection." We didn't talk on the way over. I was scared. It was just me and one officer, and I didn't know what to say to him. I liked the idea that I was getting out of juvie, but I didn't know very much about the place they were taking me.

I knew it was a mental hospital, for crazy people. That felt weird. I knew I wasn't crazy. The doctors at juvie told me I was being sent to Agnews because there wasn't anywhere else for me to go. I remember that one of them told me I might benefit from what the doctors there had to say.

I didn't hate that idea. I had liked talking to Freeman. He talked to me, and he *listened* to me, and I liked to talk to people who listened.

Just like at juvie, they put me in an observation ward for the first three weeks. I had my own room, away from the rest of the patients. It was very metallic, very utilitarian. It had a bed and a nightstand, and that was it. After lights-out, every night, they locked the door. For the first three weeks, that was my life. They took me down for a brain scan. They showed me inkblot pictures. They seemed to be studying me. All day long, day after day, I stayed in my room or sat and talked with doctors.

Life inside Agnews was very routine. Get up early. Make your bed. Breakfast in the chow hall at 5:00 AM.

Breakfast was hard-boiled eggs, sometimes oatmeal, and toast, not buttered. There was lots of coffee and lots of juice, and I liked that, and the toast was good. They baked their own bread at Agnews, and it was good bread.

After breakfast it was back to the ward. They'd hand out pills. Most of the guys were medicated. I wasn't. I was healthy. I was active—or I wanted to be. But it was hard to be active. There was a huge parkland all around us, but until you got grounds privileges you were stuck inside.

I spent most of the day walking the ward. There was a day room at one end, and a day room at the other, and a big day room in the middle. This was my world.

The day rooms were usually occupied by the worst of the mental patients. The ones who weren't in such bad shape had grounds privileges or went to work during the day. They had jobs in the kitchen, or in the bakery, making the breads and the pastries. Some guys worked in the canteen. Some guys worked on the trucks that delivered things around the place. Some guys worked on the hog farm, or had jobs with the grounds crews.

So the ones who were left behind were the ones in the worst shape—the ones who were psychotic, or catatonic, the ones who talked to themselves, or sat and drooled all day long, the ones who were unreachable.

Then there was me—the only kid in the entire facility.

Some of the patients who worked returned for lunch, which was fried baloney, or SOS—that creamed beef on toast that guys in the military love so much—or some kind of sandwich. Dinner was something similar. It was never very good. But you learned to like it or you went hungry. So I learned to like it. I learned to look forward to it.

After three weeks, the doctors took me out of the observation ward. I was given another private room. I was allowed to roam around on my own. I started figuring the place out. There seemed to be three categories of people at Agnews. First, there were the patients, who were the crazy people. Second, there were the doctors, who were supposed to be taking care of the crazy people. Third, there were the technicians, who wore all white and looked like Good Humor men. Most of them were students who were studying psychology. Their job was to keep an eye on the patients and keep them in line.

The technicians wore keys on a big key ring that jingled when they walked. You always knew when they were coming. You could hear them jingling from a mile away. They were supposed to keep an eye on us and keep us out of trouble, but they couldn't exactly sneak up on us, jingling like that. You'd hear them coming, stop what you were doing, and wait for them to go past.

I spent a lot of time talking to doctors and technicians. The doctors would bring me into their offices. The technicians would come talk to me in the day room, or during mealtime. I'd be doing a jigsaw puzzle, or trying to eat, and they'd start asking me questions. "How are you? How do you *feel*? Do you know why you're here? Do you like being here? Do you like the people here?"

I never knew what to say. I knew there were scary things going on around me. I heard stories. I knew there was electroshock. I knew there were weird medications. I didn't want anything to do with that stuff. So I tried to answer carefully. I didn't want to make anybody mad at me. I figured if I told them I thought the crazy patients were peachy keen and fine, they'd think I was crazy, too. So I told them I didn't like being around the other patients, that I was scared of what they might do to me. They seemed to understand that answer.

The patients who didn't work hung out in the day rooms. They had chairs and tables, and a TV going all the time, and you could check out stuff from an office—cards, board games, jigsaw puzzles. A lot of the guys never checked out anything. They were just *there*.

Most of them were very sick—too sick for anybody to do anything with them. Most of them were in another world. They didn't talk, except maybe to themselves. They'd just sit and rock and mutter to themselves, for hours on end. If you tried to talk to them they'd look at you like you were interrupting their conversation—with themselves. They'd wait until you left, then start talking again. I could observe them, but I couldn't really connect with them.

There were a couple of other patients I could talk to, but not many. Most of the people at Agnews weren't people I wanted to be friends with.

A lot of them were there for alcohol problems. This was before Betty Ford and all the rehab places. If a guy couldn't stop drinking, sometimes they locked him up in the nuthouse and let him dry out. There were guys like that at Agnews. Most of them were okay. They weren't crazy. They just had drinking problems.

I didn't meet any other guys who had been given lobotomies, or if I did I didn't know it. No one talked about why they were there. No one asked me. No one seemed to know what had been done to me. No one talked about what had been done to them. Being crazy wasn't something you talked about, even at a mental institution.

So I was on my own. Agnews was an adult facility, and I was the only young patient I ever saw there. That made it lonely, and strange. I didn't make friends, and I didn't have companions. But I got my own private room, and I was watched the entire time I was there. That meant I was probably safe from anything bad happening to me.

There was definitely bad stuff happening around me. You'd see guys carted off all the time. Mostly they were patients who had stopped taking their medication and had gotten violent. They'd start a fight, always with a technician. (I don't think I ever saw two patients fighting with each other.) Four or five more technicians would show up. They'd come down on the guy and haul him off to a lockup ward. It was rubber-room time.

After I had completed the so-called intake period, I was moved to a ward and finally made a friend. His name was Frank. He was Hawaiian. He was into rock 'n' roll, so we got along fine. You could check out a record player from the day room and listen to records, if you had any. Frank had good records.

I remember listening to Ritchie Valens. And Jimmy Gilmore and "Sugar Shack." And Dion and "Donna the Prima Donna." I especially liked the slow songs. I'd listen to the slow songs when I was by myself, and I'd cry inside (not boo-hoo, with tears rolling down my cheeks). I was lonely and I liked listening to songs about lonely people. *"A thousand stars in the sky/Make me realize/You are my one love . . ."* Stuff like that.

The technicians must have felt music was important. They had "music therapy" rooms they'd take the patients to. Each one had a piano or an electric organ. There were also electric guitars, and a drum set, and you could check those out. When I tried the drums, it sounded like hell. So I tried the guitar. That wasn't so bad. I had played the piano a little, and I could figure out a tune on the piano and transfer that to the guitar. I never learned to read music, because I didn't have the patience for it, but I could play a few things on the guitar.

But mostly I just listened. Here's proof of how much time I spent doing that. I figured out you could take the turntable off the record player and wrap a piece of tape around the spindle to make a 45 rpm record play slower, so that the voices were deep and low and sounded like *my* voice. That way I could sing along. After some experimenting, I found that the perfect speed for my voice was 38 rpm. I knew it was 38 rpm because I would sit, listening to the record, watching it spin around and watching the clock, and I'd actually *count* the revolutions per minute.

I had a lot of time on my hands.

I'd sit and listen to music for hours and hours, drinking coffee, smoking cigarettes, talking a little to Frank, if he was around.

Smoking was a big thing there. You spent a lot of time smoking. I had started when I was living at home, stealing Lou's cigarettes when I could, or buying a pack now and then. At Agnews, they gave the patients tobacco and papers for free. It was crummy tobacco, and crummy paper, but it was free, so that's what most of the guys smoked. You could also buy cigarettes at the canteen, and real cigarettes were like gold. If you wanted to make friends with a guy, all you needed was a pack of real cigarettes. You'd offer a guy a real cigarette and you were in.

Once I was off official observation, the doctors told me there wasn't really anything wrong with me. They told me I was okay. They told me that I didn't really *have* to be there. They said, "We don't have anyplace else to send you."

That was frustrating. I felt weird, being in a nuthouse but not being nuts. How was I going to get out? If I was crazy and I got better, they'd have to let me out. But if I wasn't crazy and I was locked up anyway, then what?

They never told me how long I was going to have to stay there.

If they had, I might have gone crazy for real. It was that kind of place. If you weren't crazy when you got there, you'd definitely be crazy when you left. Especially if you were there like I was.

Every day, I got up not knowing if today was my last day there, or whether I'd stay so long I would die there. I was just *there*, trying not to think about the past, trying not to worry about the future, trying to get through the experience one day at a time.

I lived like that, locked up at Agnews, from one day to the next, never knowing how long I was going to be there, for over a year.

My dad came to visit about twice a month. He was allowed to take me out of the ward, down to the canteen or onto the grounds. This was like a big vacation. In the whole time I was there, I never once got grounds privileges. I wasn't allowed to work on a crew, either. That meant I was locked indoors on the ward all day, every day, for the whole time. I was fourteen years old when I went in. It's hard for a fourteen-year-old kid to be locked up all day long.

So me and my dad would go down to the canteen. He was allowed to visit for an hour, or an hour and a half. He'd buy me stuff. We'd walk on the grounds, underneath those big cypress trees. He says we played tennis—I think he only says this in order to remind me that I was no good at it, and that he was frustrated by my refusal to concentrate on the game—but I don't remember that. I remember sitting in the canteen.

We talked, but we didn't talk. There was a strange silence between us. I would ask how things were going. No matter what I asked, he'd say, "Fine." I wanted to hear what was going on with George, and Brian, and Binky. I knew Binky had gotten married, and moved back into the house with his new wife. I figured George was finishing up at Covington. So I'd ask, "What's going on with Bink?" And he'd say, "He's fine," and change the subject.

My father found these visits difficult, too. He found it difficult to talk to me. He thought I was acting unhappy because I wanted to hurt him. He thought my whole attitude was one of "I'm going to make you feel bad because *I* feel bad."

I don't remember it that way. I wasn't trying to make him feel guilty. I was trying to make him love me. I felt like I had been thrown away. I wanted to know that he wanted me back again.

So, sooner or later, I would always ask him when I was going to be able to go home. And he would answer every time, "Soon." I'd ask when soon was. He'd say, "Not now. I can't take you home now."

I never asked why. I knew why. And after a while I stopped asking altogether. It was too painful to hear the answer. It hurt my feelings. It was bad to feel that unwanted. Maybe if I had been crazy, or thought I was crazy, it would have been easier. I would have known they had to keep me locked up because I wasn't right in the head. But it wasn't like that. I had to stay there because my parents didn't want me at home and no other place would take me.

So I stopped asking.

I never had any other visitors. I didn't see Lou, or my brothers. I never got any letters. Maybe that was some kind of policy, like they didn't want you to think too much about home, or else you'd run away.

I never sent any letters, either, but I wrote a lot of them. I wrote to my dad, and to Lou, and to my friends and my girlfriends. I'd tell them how much I was thinking about them, how much I was missing them, how much I loved them and cared for them, and how much I wanted to come home. I wrote letters like that to Lori, the girl whose window I broke when I was at Covington.

But I never sent any of those letters. I knew it wouldn't do any good. My dad made it clear that I wasn't going anywhere. I knew that the thing between me and Lori was over. What was I going to do, ask her to wait for me? That would not have been cool. I was in a nuthouse!

The time went slowly. It was agonizing. To make the time pass—to keep from going crazy for real—I made up stuff. I pretended. I told myself that I was in the army, like in boot camp. We were all getting ready to go overseas for the big invasion. All the other guys were going over with me. Our movements were restricted, because the invasion was top secret. I conned myself into thinking I was getting out when the invasion came—tomorrow, or the next day, or next week, but soon.

I pretended like that for the whole year I was locked up.

Freeman seemed to think Agnews was good for me. He wrote in his notes on June 7, 1963, "Howard has been at Agnews for about 3 months now. He has adjusted quite well to the hospital." I guess that meant I wasn't trying to kill myself or anybody else. Since I don't remember seeing him at Agnews, I don't know how he knew anything about it, except if Lou was making reports—and she wasn't visiting me, either. As far as he was concerned, putting me in Agnews and keeping me there was the best thing in the world for me.

Then, quite suddenly, it was over. One morning the word came that I was leaving Agnews. I was being sent to a place called Rancho Linda.

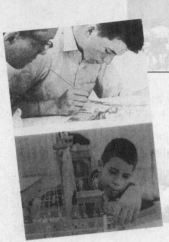

Chapter 10

Rancho Linda

Rancho Linda School sat high in the foothills to the east of San Jose. It was surrounded by fruit orchards and framed by eucalyptus trees, and it overlooked the city of San Jose and the entire Santa Clara Valley. Covering twelve acres, and built in the same low bungalow style as my elementary school and junior high school, Rancho Linda had classrooms, dormitories, dining halls, play areas, and a swimming pool. It was a privately run institution, and it had been open for less than a year when I got there.

Rancho Linda was conceived as "a residential center for special education," according to pamphlets advertising the place. It was "designed to meet the special education requirements of mentally and emotionally handicapped children and adolescents," and to deal with "educational, social and emotional deficits as they affect the learning process." The school offered "a 24-hour controlled atmosphere designed to minimize anxieties."

I am not sure whose anxieties they were designed to minimize—probably the parents', who were paying four hundred dollars a month to have their kids there—but the "24-hour controlled atmosphere" meant that Rancho Linda was a minimum security facility where the patients, or students, were kept under close watch twenty-four hours a day. There weren't bars on the windows, or armed guards, and you were allowed to roam the facilities, but it was clear that the students were confined to the compound and not expected to leave—unless they were planning to run away and never come back.

After Agnews, it felt like summer camp.

There were 110 kids there at that time, half boys, half girls, with kids as young as six and as old as seventeen or eighteen. The dorms were separated by gender and by age. There were six beds in each dorm room. Each kid had his own bed and his own closet with a clothes rack in it. Every two dorm rooms had one bathroom between them, so twelve kids shared each bathroom.

The doors were all electronically wired, and there was a big board down in the main office with lights on it that showed which doors were open (green light) and which doors were closed (red light). This was their security system. After lights-out, there was a bed check. All the doors were shut, and they were supposed to be kept shut. Sometimes there was another bed check. Sometimes the person in charge would just sit in the office looking at the big board. If all of the lights on the board were red, that meant the doors were all shut. If one of them turned green, that meant someone was leaving the room.

As a further security precaution, the dorm rooms were segregated by how difficult the kids were to handle. "D Unit" was for the bad boys. Kids would be put in there for coming to class late, for not cleaning up their rooms, for goofing around in class—stuff like that.

I spent a lot of time in D Unit.

At first I was really happy to be at Rancho Linda. The people were very friendly. The chow was incredible. Sometimes, if they didn't run out of food, you could even go back for seconds.

The classes were lame, just like most of my classes had always been, but these were extra lame. There was no algebra. There was no geometry. (To this day, I couldn't really tell you what geometry is.) There was English, and history, and art. There was music. But the classes were all too easy for me. It was like they wanted the classes to be easy so every kid could pass, so they could pat themselves on the back and say what a great job they were doing educating the kids at Rancho Linda.

I don't know what most of the other kids were doing there. With some of them, it was obvious. There were some physically handicapped kids, especially the little kids, where you could see they had leg braces or whatever. But with most of the kids, you never really knew. Some of them seemed a little slow, but there had been kids at Covington who seemed pretty slow, too. They mostly seemed like misfits, kids who couldn't get along, kids who had no place else to go.

I had no way of knowing it at the time, but some of the counselors at Rancho Linda didn't think I belonged there. One of them, a guy named Napoleon Murphy Brock, told me years later that he always thought I'd been sent there for the wrong reasons. "We didn't think there was anything really *wrong* with you," he said. "We thought the right diagnosis would have been, at most, emotionally disturbed—because of something wrong with the home environment. This was a school for mentally retarded kids, and kids with autism, and with all kinds of physical impairments. You just didn't seem to be going through the things they were going through. You didn't require the medications they required."

Because of that, maybe, Rancho Linda was an easy place for me to be successful. There were only about five cool guys in the whole school. The rest were sort of geeky. And there were about thirty girls in my age group. So it was easy for me to become one of the cool guys, right off.

For one thing, I was bigger than everybody else. I was as big as most of the counselors. Plus, I'd been around a little bit. I didn't tell people about my lobotomy, or about being at juvie, or about being at Agnews, but I knew stuff the other kids didn't know about how the world worked. Figuring out Rancho Linda was a snap.

A brochure from the early Rancho Linda days promised "off-campus events including fairs, rodeos, beach parties, professional sports events, bowling, movies, plays, visits to industrial plants, public recreation areas, zoos, ranches, government and armed forces facilities." Students would participate in "swim meets, intramural games, hikes, picnics and Friday night dances."

I remember the occasional dance, but I don't remember doing many other things from that list. We did get taken down the hill sometimes to a place called the What's It Club in Santa Clara, which was run by an ex-policeman who was friends with one of the counselors. It was a drinking place, except when we were there. For us, it was just sodas and dancing.

So there wasn't a lot you could do for fun at Rancho Linda. We took hikes in the hills around the school. There was a running team, and I ran cross-country, but I don't remember us ever competing against another school. There was the swimming pool. But there wasn't much to actually *do*.

So that left smoking and sex. Those were the two things you weren't supposed to do, and we all wanted to do them. I figured out how to do them both.

Getting cigarettes wasn't that hard. There was one girl at the school who was old enough to smoke, and her parents would bring her cigarettes. We'd steal them from her, or she would give them to us. There was one counselor who, if he had to drive you down the hill to go to a doctor's appointment or dentist appointment, would let you buy cigarettes. There was another counselor who left cigarettes in her car, unlocked, all the time. I think she was leaving them there for us, because it was almost always a full pack, and we'd take it one day and there'd be a fresh pack there the next day.

You weren't allowed to smoke at the school. You especially weren't allowed to smoke in the dorms. But that's what we did. We'd open a window and smoke standing next to it, blowing the smoke out. Every once in a while we'd hear one of the night counselors coming and we'd throw our cigarettes out the window and jump back in bed. There was one counselor, a Japanese guy named Yamaguchi, who'd stick his head in the door. The room would be *full* of smoke. He'd say, "You boys not been smoking in here?" And we'd say, "Oh, no, Mr. Yamaguchi, not us." And he'd leave us alone.

Standing by the window and smoking got me thinking: *If no one catches me smoking by the window, I bet no one would catch me sneaking out the room by the window, either.* So one night I popped the screen and climbed outside. The windows were not wired like the doors were. No one knew I had left the room. So I wandered around. The next day, I told one of the girls I might be coming by for a visit.

By the time I figured out how to escape the dorm at night, I had already been fooling around with girls at Rancho Linda. I had been with a girl named Susan. She had a big bust and, like a lot of the girls at that time, wore her hair bobbed, like a backup singer from The Ronettes or some band like that. She was aggressive, and she was easy, and I'd be lying if I said there was any other reason I went with her. She made it happen. But she didn't really know *how* to make it happen, and neither did I. So we didn't really have intercourse. We did a lot of making out, but we didn't go all the way.

For that, I had to wait for Annette.

I had a real crush on her. She wasn't like Susan. She was something special. She was very bubbly and outgoing, and cute. Some guys might have said she was a little heavier than she should be, but not me. I always liked girls with a little meat on their bones, and she had that.

I don't know what she was doing at Rancho Linda. There certainly didn't seem to be anything wrong with her. Maybe she was a discipline problem at home. Maybe she was like me, and no one knew where to put her. I never asked. Just like at Agnews, no one at Rancho Linda ever asked.

I wanted her so badly. I didn't know what to do about that, any more than I did with Susan, but Annette was so beautiful that I was willing to make a complete fool of myself trying if I ever got the chance. Then I got the chance.

The first time it happened, I was lying in bed pretending to be sick. The other kids were in school. I didn't want to go. So I faked sick. While the other kids were in class, I was alone in my room.

Annette heard I was sick, and she came down to see how I was doing. She got a bathroom pass or something, and snuck down to visit me.

I was scared to death. I was really into Annette. Plus, I didn't want to get caught. I was already on D Unit. You couldn't go anywhere from there but out. I didn't want to get into trouble. And I was scared of what I imagined we were about to do. I was afraid she would see that I didn't know what I was doing. I was afraid I'd look like a nerd.

We had already hugged and kissed and messed around a little, but I didn't really know how to go any further. I'm not sure Annette really knew, either.

But we were alone and we had time. Annette got into bed with me. We had thirty minutes together before she had to leave. Somehow we figured it out. I don't know if Annette was a virgin before that day. But neither one of us was afterward.

It was wonderful. It was so exciting. I felt like a man. I felt like I had crossed over. I wasn't a kid anymore.

I knew the word was going to get out. I wasn't going to tell anyone—I knew that you didn't do that, and besides, I didn't want to get caught. But I thought Annette would tell her friends.

She told. Within a day, the other girls knew what had happened. Pretty soon some of the guys knew, too. Now I could walk around like I owned the place. I had arrived.

Then, almost as fast, I had a big scare. Annette was pregnant. First she told all her friends what had happened. Then she started saying she was pregnant.

I knew it had to be me, because she hadn't been with anybody else. But I also couldn't figure out how it was possible. I mean, we were together one time. How could she get pregnant? Also, how could she be so sure so soon? It had only been about three days. Could a girl know she was pregnant in three days?

That shows you how much I knew. Of course it turned out she wasn't pregnant, and everything was fine.

These escapades became my big thing. Every night I was on a

Mission: Impossible kind of mission—to bust out of my room and sneak up to one of the girls' dorms.

After dark, after the bed check, I would take the screen off the window in my room and crawl outside. I'd sneak across the campus. Then I'd usually have to climb a fence, or climb the side of the building and crawl along the roof, to get to the girls' dorm.

I took it seriously. I'd even wear dark clothing in order to blend in with the surroundings. Sometimes I'd hear someone coming, and I'd have to lie down and hide. One night I heard footsteps so close to me that I knew I was busted. I hit the deck and lay in the gravel, and waited for what seemed like forever. Then the footsteps went away.

That's the way it was at Rancho Linda. And it wasn't just me. I don't know if I was the first guy to bust out and go visit the girls, but I wasn't the last. Pretty soon it seemed liked everybody was doing it. We all had our schemes. To get around the bed checks, you'd roll up a bunch of clothes and stick them under your sheets. Then you'd slip out. The bed checks never came more often than thirty minutes apart, so you knew you had a half hour to take care of business. Sometimes you'd sneak out and get up to the girls' room and be back in fifteen minutes. Sometimes it was an aborted mission—when you got out and found someone patrolling outside. Or you'd get to the girls' room and open a screen and someone would scream. Or you'd find the window locked.

We were successful a lot of the time, I think, because Rancho Linda was a new facility with a young, inexperienced staff. They hadn't figured out yet what we would be up to, so they hadn't figured out how to stop us.

I went up to Annette's room the first time maybe a month after our first experience together. Then word got around that I was in the know as far as the sex thing went. So pretty soon there were these other girls paying attention to me. Susan was interested in me again. So was Cindy. She was a very aggressive girl. Some people said she was a slut. They called her a whore. So, it wasn't good to be caught with Cindy. But it was very good to be *alone* with Cindy.

Annette found out these other girls were interested in me. She got jealous and broke up with me. So, I was with Susan for a while. Then Susan found out I was interested in Cindy, so she wouldn't have anything to do with me for a while. And so it went. I guess I thought I was a stud. What did I know?

I made friends with a guy named Ron. He was cool. He was Latin, and he had a waterfall haircut. He might have been at Rancho Linda for physical problems. He had a bad arm—one arm didn't work right. And we had gotten to be friends in a weird way. We were playing around and I pushed him down and hurt his leg. We weren't playing that hard, so I didn't know why it hurt him. But he went to the nurse, and he wound up in the hospital. It turned out he had some kind of weird bone infection. That's why his leg hurt when I pushed him down. They said if he hadn't found out about the infection when he did, he would have lost the leg.

After he got better, Ron and I started going up to the girls' dorm together. He became my partner in crime. We'd sneak out and go up there. He had a bunch of girls, like I did.

He wasn't my only friend. I also got to be friends with a whole bunch of other guys. We had some good times together—and not just with the girls. We pulled some pranks. One time we figured out that four of us, working together, could pick up a Volkswagen. So we did. We picked one up out of the parking lot and carried it down the driveway, and set it sideways so cars couldn't pass. I don't know if they ever figured out who did that, or how.

The counselors and administrators had this attitude that they didn't want their school to be a prison. So there were no bars on the windows, and the doors were not locked, even if they were monitored. So we snuck around a lot. We'd sneak into the kitchen and make sandwiches and bring them back to our beds. I found out you could use a butter knife to break into the Coke machine, so we all had Cokes with our sandwiches.

Remember, a lot of us were troublemakers before we got to Rancho Linda. So a lot of us continued to be troublemakers while we were there.

I was often homesick. My dad would visit every few weeks. We'd take a walk, or we'd sit and have coffee in the cafeteria. He would ask me about the school. I'd tell him about what went on there—not everything, but some of it. He was critical of the school. He was spending money out of his own pocket to keep me there. Even though I was still a ward of the court, some of the expense came directly from home. There was an official Rancho Linda clothing list, and the family had to buy everything on it. And then the clothing would get lost or damaged in the laundry, and the shirt or the pants or something would have to be replaced. It burned my dad up to spend money on things like that. He was raising three other boys at home, and money didn't grow on trees—even in Los Altos.

In the beginning, like at Agnews, I'd ask my dad when he was going to take me home. For a while, he'd say, "Well, maybe pretty soon," or, "Well, this isn't really a good time," or, "We'll have to wait and see." Sometimes he'd just say, "Not now." I got the idea that he didn't want me asking the question anymore, so again I stopped asking.

Lou came to visit once. Just once. I was actually happy to see her. I jumped up and tried to give her a hug and a kiss. She pushed me away. She didn't say anything, but nothing had changed. She didn't want anything to do with me.

It hurt me. The funny thing is, even after everything that had happened, I wanted to love her and I wanted her to love me. I wanted a mother, even if it was Lou. I didn't want to be this angry rebel kid who was locked up because no one could handle him. I wanted to be a normal kid who lived at home with his mom and dad and brothers, who went to school and did all the normal kid stuff. Even after everything that had happened, I still wished I had that kind of family.

There were things about Rancho Linda that made me less lonely and homesick, like having a girlfriend, or hanging out with Ron or the other guys I was friends with. But there were things about Rancho Linda that made me more lonely and homesick.

For one thing, the school sat on this hill, way high up, but still close enough to the suburbs that you could see what was going on down there. You could see downtown San Jose from the classrooms. You could see the neon lights showing where the movie theaters were. You could see other schools. You could see kids playing on school playgrounds. If you were in the yard in front of the school, you could actually *hear* the kids playing. You could see kids riding their bikes in front of their houses. You could see dads coming home from work in the evening.

I spent a lot of time in that front yard, because that's where you got sent when you were being punished. You'd get sentenced to two days of weeding, and for the next two afternoons you'd be out there pulling weeds in the sun, looking down the hill and hearing the voices of the kids at the normal school, with the normal lives.

I got punished a lot. Things weren't that strict at Rancho Linda, but there were rules, and I had a hard time not breaking the rules. Some of the rules were stupid. You'd get in trouble for coming to class late, or goofing off in class, or being disruptive. You'd get in trouble for little things, too. One time I got in trouble for not making my bed before breakfast.

There were these male counselors. Some of them were students from San Jose State. Some of them were studying to be doctors. Some of them were just people who needed a job. Some of them were cool, and some of them were not.

One of them was named Billy Cooper. He was a black guy from San Jose State. He wore sharkskin suits and was always flirting with the ladies—the other counselors, and even the students. He was cool.

Another was Napoleon Murphy Brock, the counselor I spoke to years after I left Rancho Linda. He was black, too, and he was a musician. He played all kinds of instruments. He was studying psychology and music at San Jose State. A few years after I knew him, he was hired by Frank Zappa to join his band, The Mothers of Invention. (He still tours today with Frank's son Dweezil.) He was cool.

Another was an ex–Olympic boxer named Lou Rawls, just like the singer. He wasn't too bad.

Another was Frank Schuler. He was German. He had also been an Olympic athlete, a fast walker, back in Germany. He was tough. He would make you run around the basketball courts for hours as punishment. He'd make you stand outside with your hands outstretched. You couldn't move them. After twenty or thirty minutes that is hard to do, and it hurts. He was *not* cool.

Worst of all was a redheaded guy named Doug.

One morning Doug stopped me on the way to breakfast and told me I had to make my bed. I didn't want to. I wanted breakfast. I was hungry. But he stopped me and said I wasn't leaving until I made my bed.

It wasn't the first time we'd had a problem. He was always ragging me, telling me he was going to teach me a lesson or straighten me out. So this time I said, "Go ahead. Right here."

We started fighting, and I got him in a headlock, and then I started punching him in the face. That's how the other counselors found us.

Lou Rawls was the administrator that day. He took me and Doug down to this exercise room where there was a sort of boxing ring. He made us put on boxing gloves—just like Lou did years before with me and George—and told us to get in there and settle our differences like men.

It didn't last long. Doug charged me and I hit him in the stomach. He went down. And even though this was supposed to be a private thing, there was a cheer from a bunch of students who had gathered outside the window and seen me knock Doug down.

Lou Rawls took Doug out of the ring, and put the gloves on Frank Schuler. I think he wanted me to learn a lesson, and the lesson wasn't supposed to be me beating up Doug inside the ring *and* outside the ring. So I had to go a few rounds with Schuler. Unfortunately he was a better fighter than Doug. He knocked me down once, and I got up. He knocked me down a second time, and I got up again. But the third time he knocked me down, I decided to stay down. I wasn't stupid. I stayed on the ground.

That made Schuler mad. He started yelling at me, and then he kicked me. Lou Rawls jumped in and stopped the fight. He said if he ever saw Schuler kick another man when he was down, he'd put on the gloves and show him what real fighting was.

Lou Rawls was an ex-boxer. You didn't want to mess with him. It impressed me that he stood up for me that way, and Schuler backed down at once.

I don't remember being very unhappy at Rancho Linda. Not happy, either, but not miserable. I had the thing going with Annette. That was important to me. I guess I was in love with her. I certainly thought about her all the time. I never thought about being with other girls when I could be with her.

But we never talked about the future. We never talked about what would happen when we got out of Rancho Linda. I don't know if that's being a teenager, or being a teenager in a place like Rancho Linda, but you lived only for the day, or only for the moment. It was all about getting through whatever was happening *right now*. You didn't worry too much about what was coming later, because right now was all you could deal with.

It was like you were in a river, caught in the current, and you were going whatever way it took you. You knew you had no control over your own destiny. So you didn't dream, and you didn't plan. There was no reason to plan. You knew you had to survive what you were going through, and the way to make it survivable was to try to have fun.

I had some fun. My dad bought me an electric guitar, a Fender copy that came from Sears. I *loved* that guitar. I played it for hours and hours. I was really into music. I didn't perform, and I didn't want to perform, even though I fantasized about being a pop star. I would sing to myself, in my room, for hours, but I would never sing in public. I didn't have the voice for it, and I knew it. But when I was alone, I was Paul Anka and I sang beautifully.

There was real music at Rancho Linda sometimes. One of the directors of the school knew Connie Stevens, the singer. The director's name was Stevens, and he said he was her cousin or something. I don't think he was. Connie Stevens is Italian, and her real name isn't even Stevens. But he knew her, and he somehow got her to come and perform at Rancho Linda. It's funny that I don't remember what songs she sang, because it was a pretty big thing. She had starred on the TV detective show *Hawaiian Eye*, and she had a big radio hit with Edd "Kookie" Byrnes, called "Kookie, Kookie (Lend Me Your Comb)," after Edd became a star on *77 Sunset Strip*. I don't remember if she sang that, but I do remember she was beautiful, and I got her autograph.

Sometimes the fun we had was at the expense of someone else. We used to make fun of some of the kids, or tease them, or even bully them. George Pezzolo, for example, had a stamp collection— a huge stamp collection. He kept it hidden in his room, but everyone knew where it was. It was very precious to him. Sometimes when he was being obnoxious I'd tell him I was going to go get his stamp collection and make paper airplanes out of it. He'd get upset and tell the teacher, and the teacher would let him go back to his room to guard his stamp collection. We teased him so much that in the end, he built this huge wooden box, with a big lock on it, big enough to hold his entire stamp collection. He carried it around with him all the time, because he thought we were going to break into it.

Other guys, if they gave us too much difficulty, we'd have a "blanket party" for them. We'd wait for the guy to come into one of the bedrooms. Then we'd throw a blanket over his head and beat him. We never *really* hurt anyone. We never sent anyone to the hospital, or even to the nurse. But we must have scared some guys pretty bad.

This was my life. I grew up a little. I got taller. I felt a little more like a man. There's a picture of me from that period at a Friday night dance, in the Rancho Linda courtyard, dancing with Annette. I'm wearing a sport coat, and I'm about four feet taller than her. She has a dress on, and her hair is up, and we look good together.

Eventually, I got bored enough to get into some real trouble. That's what happened with my big plan for the prison break.

Like I've already said, I was a big fan of the TV show *Mission: Impossible.* I can hear that theme music now, and I can remember dreaming about having those kinds of top-secret adventures myself. So, I invented one.

I created this plan to take over Rancho Linda and make an escape. I started drawing up plans. I sketched a blueprint of the dormitory and the administration building. I figured out how we could overpower the counselors. We would take the wooden curtain rods out of our closets, and use them to club the counselors into submission. We'd tie them up, the ones in the boys' dorm and the ones in the girls' dorm. Then we'd bust out. Everyone was going to escape.

Except me. I had a *secret* secret plan. The other guys would bust out, but I would stay behind with the girls who didn't want to go. I would have them all to myself.

I was never serious about this plan. It was just a goof. But once the other guys found out about it, it got serious. They thought it was a real plan. I couldn't tell them it was all a joke, or I'd look like an idiot. So I let them think it was real, even though I never thought it was.

We drew up plans. I had them hidden under my mattress. We picked a night, and the night was approaching. We all had our instructions. This kid was going to be posted here, and this kid was going to be posted there. Everyone had his job. It would be just like the TV show. "Your mission, should you choose to accept it . . ."

Then one of the kids snitched. We got called on the carpet by the administrators. They knew the whole plan. They knew the date. They knew the details. They hadn't found the plans, though, and they didn't know who the ringleader was. But they knew who was involved, and they were going to throw the book at the whole bunch of us.

So I stepped forward and admitted I was behind the whole thing. I didn't want to do that, but I also didn't want the whole school to go down because of me.

I got three weeks of pulling weeds on the front hill. Some of the other guys got two weeks, or one week. But I got three—since I was the brains behind the operation!

I wanted to tell them it was all a joke, but I couldn't risk looking bad in front of the whole school. It would be better to take the three weeks and look like I was cool.

Since they didn't know it was a joke, the administrators didn't know it wouldn't happen again. They had the cops positioned outside the school for several weeks after that. Night after night, we'd see them walking the grounds, standing outside our windows, wearing their SWAT-type gear, waiting for the riot that never came.

That was the summer of 1965, I think. I was a tough guy. I was sixteen and a half years old.

During my time at the school, I didn't see too much of Freeman. According to his notes, he came to visit me once. I don't remember it, but he wrote it up for his files.

"I saw Howard this evening at Rancho Linda School," Freeman wrote on April 23, 1964.

> *He is certainly the tallest and, maybe, one of the older among the boys. It is said that he is making very good progress in the matter of self control and keeping the younger boys in line. He is visited by his father and step-mother about every week, but seldom gets home. There has been a big change in the home situation . . . since, now that Howard is out of the picture, his dis-*

ruptive influence has allowed the family to come back together. The older boy is doing much better work in school and the younger boy has stopped wetting his bed and having nightmares. Mr. and Mrs. Dully seem to be getting along much more peaceably than they were.

Lou visited Freeman in October, 1965. He wrote,

Mrs. Dully tells me that Howard is now 6'4", a regular bean pole, two inches taller than her husband, and has not been home since Christmas time which was pretty upsetting to him and to the family. He is to be allowed out for November 24 and 25. His father goes to see him twice a month on visiting days, and his reports are pretty good, although sometimes he is marked down for his deportment. His latest desire is to get more English— ordinarily, Howard could not care less. He spends a good deal of time in his dormitory [where] his formidable size makes it easy for him to become somewhat of a peace keeper. He has had no convulsions. He eats and sleeps well. Howard says he likes it at school and wants to stay there.

I guess I would have stayed there, too, at least until I finished high school. But something happened and Rancho Linda ended just like *that*.

One morning I was getting ready for breakfast when a counselor came into the room. He said, "Pack your stuff. You're leaving."

I didn't find out right away what had happened. I was too busy worrying about me. What was going to happen to me? Where was I going? Home? If not home, where? I packed my stuff and waited.

What happened was, after all the nightly dorm visits, someone had snitched. One of the girls had complained. Maybe she told her family. Maybe her family told the school officials—or threatened to make an official complaint. Either way, some students were caught having sex in the dorms.

It turned into a big story. The headline from one San Jose paper read, SEX PARTY AT SCHOOL—FOUR HELD. The headline from another paper read, EIGHT HELD FOLLOWING RANCHO LINDA "ORGY." The details were the same, except for the number.

"Four teenage couples were booked at Juvenile Hall yesterday in the wake of what sheriff's investigators called a sex party in the girls' dormitory at the Rancho Linda school for disturbed children," the second account said. "The four boys and four girls range from 13 to 17 years old.

"Officers said the boys climbed in a window of the dormitory. . . . The party broke up when a counselor discovered the couples in bed. Three of the girls admitted having sexual relations with their partners."

That was March 10, 1966. On March 22, 1966, it was over. JUVENILE SCHOOL GIVES UP LICENSE AFTER SEX PARTY, the headline read.

"Rancho Linda School, where authorities reportedly discovered a teenage sex party in a girls' dormitory two weeks ago, voluntarily has surrendered its license to the State Department of Mental Hygiene and today has transferred all but seven of its 150 wards to other institutions."

I think the counselors may have known all along that some of the kids were messing around. They certainly had known something was going on with me and Annette. They had fun with it. One time I was sick in bed with tonsillitis and a high fever. I couldn't get up to eat my meals, so they sent Annette down with my dinner on a tray. It was torture! We were alone, but we couldn't do anything. In the end, though, the joke was on them. My fever broke and I felt much better, but I didn't tell anyone. They kept sending Annette down with that tray, but now I was feeling good enough to do something when she got there.

I never found out who snitched, or got caught, but I heard later that thirty of the thirty-two teenage girls at Rancho Linda were discovered to be pregnant. At the time, all I could think was, *How did we miss those two?*

But it was no joke. Rancho Linda was the best thing that had happened to me for a while, and I had no idea how much I would miss it after it was gone.

The next thing I knew, I was back in juvie.

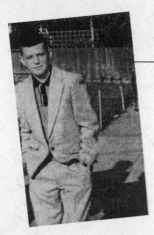

Chapter 11

Agnews. Again.

They couldn't keep me in Juvenile Hall. I hadn't committed any crime—I wasn't even one of the guys they caught in bed at Rancho Linda. I hadn't been accused of anything. Besides, I was barely even a juvenile anymore. It was April 1966. I was seventeen and a half years old. I was practically grown up.

I was tall enough and big enough—six feet four inches and probably about 180 pounds. I had done enough sports at Rancho Linda that I was physically fit—no Jack LaLanne, but I was in good shape. In the pictures that I have from that time, I see a clean-cut guy who wears his hair short and his sport coat tight and has a little bit of an attitude. In most of the pictures from this period, I've got a smirk. Not quite a smile. Not quite a frown. Just a sort of look that says, "I know what a joke this all is."

It seemed like a joke. It was like my dream of being in the army had come true. Now I had done my time in the service, and I was furloughed out. I was being returned to civilian life, and would walk the streets again with the rest of the citizens.

But I couldn't go home. Despite Freeman's reports about my continued progress, and the fact that I'd gotten through a few years at Rancho Linda without killing anybody, I was not welcome at the house on Edgewood. Lou still wouldn't have me.

So, after a short stay at juvie, I was placed in a halfway house with a collection of other misfit guys who, like me, didn't have anyplace else to go. The house was a two-story stucco with a glassed-in front porch and a kind of Oriental wood trim. The corners of the roof turned up like a pagoda. The address was 619 North First Street in San Jose.

The place was run by a crabby old lady. She fixed our meals and made sure the rules were followed. But there weren't many rules. You had to be out by a certain time in the morning, and you had to be back by a certain time at night. Your rent was paid by the government, directly to the old lady. You got a little allowance out of that, so you could buy cigarettes and coffee. (I smoked Marlboro reds in those days.) Other than that, it didn't matter what you did with yourself as long as you stayed out of trouble.

I did, for a while. Someone from the Welfare Department or the Probation Department or Social Services arranged a little job for me with Goodwill Industries. They called it a job, but it was a joke. I was paid ten cents an hour to sort through boxes of clothes. Ten cents an hour! Even for a guy with no work experience, that was insulting. The minimum wage was something like $1.25 or $1.35. How did they get away with paying someone ten cents an hour? In my case, they didn't—not for long. I stopped going to work.

There was an International House of Pancakes right down the block. I'd go down there and hang out and drink coffee and talk to the people I'd meet. I fell in with some bad characters. I met a group of guys who belonged to this motorcycle gang called the Gypsy Jokers. They had names like Shorty and Butcher. They were like the Hells Angels, but maybe not as dangerous, and they let me hang out with them. Since I didn't have a bike and wasn't going to ride with them, they didn't have to jump me in or do any of that hairy initiation stuff. They just let me hang out. They all drank at this beer bar called The Spartan Hub. In the afternoons and evenings, when I wasn't busy goofing off at the IHOP, I'd go down there and drink beer with them. I thought I was pretty cool—not even eighteen yet, and here I was drinking beer with the Gypsy Jokers.

Back at the halfway house I made friends with a guy named Ed Woodson. He was a skinny little guy who wore a beard and mustache over what I think was a cleft palate. He had a slight speech impediment, and a weird habit of saying "But one thing" whenever he had something to say. He said it like he was sharing a secret, or like he was afraid you were going to get mad at him, but it was meaningless. You'd ask him if he wanted to go downtown. He'd lean over and say, "Yeah, but one thing: I have to go see my probation officer. . . ."

I never knew what his background was or how he wound up in the halfway house, but we got to be buddies and started having some fun together. Sometimes the fun backfired, which seemed to happen a lot with me.

Usually it started out sort of innocent. There was a guy at the halfway house who had a motorcycle. He thought he was so cool, with his little motorcycle. We were jealous, so we decided to teach him a lesson.

I got two paper milk containers, one empty and one full. I drained the gas out of his tank into the empty one, and then I filled the gas tank with milk from the full one. I hid the two milk containers in the rubbish pit. We sat back to see what would happen to the guy's bike.

That wasn't very dramatic. The bike just wouldn't start. The guy looked in the gas tank and saw this milky stuff and could not figure out what the heck had happened. It was pretty funny.

It wasn't so funny the next time the gardener went out to the rubbish pit. He took the rubbish and put it in the incinerator, and started a fire. The gas ignited, and the milk container exploded. The whole backyard went up in flames, and the house almost burned down.

I didn't get caught for that one.

Ed Woodson was a bit wilder than me. He had more experience. He knew people. For example, he knew two guys who had escaped from the county jail. I don't know how they got out. I don't know how Ed knew them. But when they escaped, they came straight to the halfway house. Ed hid them in the basement and snuck food down to them for a few days. When the heat was off, they left. I thought that was wild. Guys escaping from jail! Hiding out in our basement! It was like James Cagney and Edward G. Robinson. This was the big time.

I didn't get caught for that one, either. Ed didn't get caught. I don't know whether the two guys went back to jail or what. At the time, I didn't even realize it was serious.

And that was part of the problem. I didn't understand what was serious and what wasn't. I knew the difference between right and wrong. But I didn't really understand the significance of *doing* right and wrong. I had no idea how to behave. I was on the street, and I had all this freedom, but I had no idea what to do with it.

For example . . .

Ever since Rancho Linda, I had been thinking about Annette. She had been my special girl. I kept with me a picture of the two of us dancing. She had written on the back of it, "For Howard, from Annette. I hope one day to be your wife."

I heard she was staying with some friends, or some family member, in Glendale, a San Fernando Valley suburb of Los Angeles. Ed Woodson had family in Los Angeles somewhere. We decided we'd hitchhike down there together. I'd surprise Annette and he'd surprise his family.

We set out like it was going to be a little overnight visit. We didn't have much money. We didn't have any gear—nothing to eat, nothing to sleep on, nothing to wash with, nothing but the clothes on our backs.

It took us a long time to get to Los Angeles. A trucker picked us up and left us out in the sticks. We stood on the side of the highway all night trying to get a lift. It took three days just to get down to Ventura.

We split up there. Ed went on to Los Angeles. I went into the San Fernando Valley. I don't remember where my last ride dropped me off, but I walked the rest of the way. The area was mostly orange groves in those days, and dirt roads. I walked for an entire day, down these dusty dirt roads, eating oranges the whole time, until I got to Glendale.

I hadn't written to Annette to tell her I was coming. Now I knocked on the door. Some guy came out and said she wasn't home. He said she might be back later. I said thank you and I left.

I was crushed. I had left San Jose with very little money. Now I didn't have a dime. I had hardly eaten, except for those oranges, in a couple of days. I hadn't bathed or changed clothes since leaving the halfway house. I was filthy. I was scared, too.

So I got mad. How dare Annette not be at home! What a nerve! Didn't she know I had practically walked across the state of California to see her? Didn't she love me anymore?

I suppose I could have waited for her. I could have asked her family to let me come in and wait for her. But I didn't. I don't remember whether I even thought about those things. Probably I wasn't thinking too clearly. I was tired and hungry and upset. I probably wasn't thinking at all. So I went back out to the highway and started hitchhiking.

I don't remember how long it took, but I found myself in King City, California, up in the Central Valley. And there, hitching on the side of the road, I bumped into Ed. He had been hitching awhile, and he wasn't getting any rides, so he was going to buy a bus ticket home. When he saw me, though, he changed his mind. We used his money to buy some food, and then we hitchhiked back to San Jose.

I never saw Annette again. I didn't write. I have no idea what happened to her. I don't know whether she ever knew that the dirty, crazy nut who came to her door that day was me.

For some reason I didn't get into trouble for being away from the halfway house for those few days. The crabby old lady let me and Ed in, and we went back to our old routine. It wasn't much of a routine. It wasn't much of a life.

I was nearly eighteen. I was old enough to be doing all kinds of things. But I didn't really know *how* to do anything. I didn't have a high school diploma. I had never applied for a job. I didn't have a checking account or a savings account. I had no idea how to handle money. I had never washed my own clothes. I didn't know how to cook for myself—even though I had helped out in the kitchen at Rancho Linda sometimes. I had never bought food for myself in a grocery store. I had never bought myself a pair of pants or a shirt or a pair of shoes. I had never gotten myself a haircut. I had no idea how to do *anything*.

But now, out on the street, I was expected to take care of myself and stay out of trouble. I wasn't very good at taking care of myself. My size usually kept bad guys away from me. I looked like I was going to be a problem. But if someone did come after me, I really didn't know what to do about it.

Living on First Street, I was attacked one night. I was on the street in front of the halfway house and this guy sprang up out of nowhere and pulled a knife on me. He grabbed me by the hair—I had really long hair at the time—and said he was going to chop all my hair off.

I didn't know what to do, but I was scared, so I started screaming. That was the right thing to do. He ran away without cutting my hair off, and he didn't come back.

The real trouble I got into was of my own making.

One day me and Ed were sitting at the halfway house when the mail came. There was a bank statement in there, delivered to the wrong address, with a bunch of canceled checks from the IRS. I guess they were refund checks. They were in large amounts, like $1,000 and $1,500. They were canceled, but the bank mark showing the cancelations was so light that you could rub it out with an eraser without damaging the paper. So I hatched a plan.

I'd take the check to a bank and open a checking account. I'd say I wanted to deposit the $1,000, and have $200 in cash. Then I'd get a pack of temporary checks until my own personal checks could be printed. I'd leave the bank with money in my pocket and a handful of temporary checks.

I didn't know if it would work. The IRS checks were no good, because they'd already been cashed, but the bank might not know that for a couple of days. By then, I'd pull the same thing with another check at another bank.

Meanwhile I started visiting pawnshops. I'd look around until I decided I wanted to buy something like an electric guitar. Actually, I *did* want to buy it. It was a nice guitar. But that wasn't the idea. The guitar cost, say, three hundred dollars. I paid for it with a bad check. Then I took the guitar across town to another pawnshop. I hocked it for maybe a hundred bucks. *That* was the idea.

It was the perfect crime. Suddenly I was rich. I had a hundred bucks in cash, plus what I'd gotten from the bank. This was more money than I'd ever had in my life. I didn't even know what to do with all the money. I'd hail a cab and ride around for half the night, just to spend a few bucks.

It was a great scam. Since it worked once, I figured it would work again. I did the same scam several times, buying things at one pawnshop with a bad check, then taking them to another pawnshop and hocking them there. I raised some good money that way.

The problem was this: I was a bad criminal. I had criminal instincts, but not a criminal mind. When you write a blank check at a place like a pawnshop, the pawnshop owner asks you for your name and address and phone number. Since it was a fake account and I didn't have any money, I didn't think it mattered what name and address I gave him. So I wrote down my right name, and I wrote down the address and phone number of the halfway house.

The phone calls started coming in. The checks were no good. The banks were onto me. The pawnshop guys knew where I was. It was only a matter of time before someone came to get me.

A real criminal would have run away. I didn't. I just waited.

The call came from a Lieutenant Lance Hunt. He explained to me that I was in some trouble, and that the trouble would be worse if I tried to run from it. He said that he was coming over to get me, and that I'd better be there.

I waited.

Despite my little bits of trouble in the past, this was my first serious contact with the law. Before, I had just been a screw-up. Now

I was a criminal. I had committed a felony. Passing bad checks was a serious crime. I guess I knew that, but I didn't really calculate what kind of trouble I'd be in if they caught me.

Well, they caught me. And I found out pretty quickly what kind of trouble I was in. They told me guys went to prison for this kind of thing, even guys who were only seventeen and a half years old. Guys went to prison for one to fourteen years.

I was fingerprinted. They took my mug shot. They took away my belt and my shoelaces. They stuck me in a cell.

At some point while I was in Agnews or at Rancho Linda, my dad had gotten interested in law enforcement. He had become a reserve deputy sheriff. Over the years he had worked at the jail, helped the sheriff's department with transportation, done court security as a bailiff, and helped train other reserve officers. He had never been an actual policeman, but he knew lots of cops.

He must have known someone in the San Jose Police Department, because they contacted my dad and talked to him about my situation. They offered him some sort of deal.

My dad came to tell me the details. The cops had agreed to let me off the hook. No prison time. No jail time. All I had to do was let them stick me back in Agnews for a while. If I could convince the people at Agnews that I was a little bit crazy, I could stay there instead of going to jail. He made it real clear to me that if I didn't convince them I was crazy, I was going to jail. Or, worse than jail, I would go to prison.

I didn't know what prison was like. But I had been to Juvenile Hall, and county jail, and I could imagine. I didn't want to go there. Oh, boy, did I *not* want to go there. So I made the deal. I agreed to go back to Agnews and act crazy.

Someone got the word to Freeman.

"Howard has been readmitted to Agnews in the last few days," the doctor wrote on September 23, 1966.

The Rancho School has closed down when it was discovered that the patients were enjoying too much sexual freedom, and Howard was at some halfway house where he adjusted pretty well until he got hold of a batch of checks and made out a number of them to his friends and others until the law caught up with him. Both his mother and father were very much concerned over the possibility of his coming back into the home, saying that his influence would be definitely disrupting. They arranged for his commitment.

The following day, Freeman came for a visit.

I saw Howard at Agnews today on the admission ward where he was sent from jail after a bad check. He says he has not been home at all, but has been living in San Jose in a house with other discharged patients. He was employed for several weeks at Good Will sorting cards at 10 cents an hour, which he said was not enough to buy his cigarettes, so he got disgusted and quit. Then he found out that people were getting 60 cents an hour, so he was disgruntled. "I like it better in here than out there." Howard has filled out quite a bit and is, I think, at least as tall as his father. He talks fairly freely, and in the few minutes I had with him did not express any unusual ideas.

I was saving my unusual ideas for the Agnews staff. My dad had told me that I had to convince them I was a little nutty in order to stay there, and out of jail. So I tried to look a little nutty.

At the beginning I was on the observation ward. But I was on a tighter rein this time. The doctors needed to come up with a report. The court people and the probation people had to make a recommendation. So they were watching me closely. They had to gather all the data on me.

I gave it my best shot. I tried to show them I was crazy. It was just a matter of acting weird at the right times. Anyone can do that. You don't have to be crazy to act crazy. You just have to know what crazy people act like. And I had plenty of experience watching crazy people.

Crazy people hit themselves. They talk to themselves. So, I

did that. I don't know how convincing I was, especially with the talking-to-myself part. I thought it was stupid, and I thought I looked stupid doing it. But if they were looking for something to write about, I was going to give it to them. I was going to make them say, "Okay, this guy's a nut."

I talked to myself about normal things, just like I was telling a friend a story. But I also invented things. Like, I invented a guitar and amplifier that didn't exist. One of the techs would come to talk to me. I'd see him coming and I'd start talking to myself. Then he'd start to sit in a chair and I'd say, "Hey! Watch out. That's my guitar and amp there!"

That seemed to make them pick up their notebooks pretty fast.

My crazy act worked. I made the doctors think that I needed to be there. After three weeks or so, they made their recommendation, and I was allowed to stay. I was allowed to not go to prison.

I guess I figured that once they knew about the lobotomy, the doctors and technicians would give me a break. The funny thing is, it never occurred to me that if I convinced them I was crazy, I would have trouble convincing them later on that I was *not* crazy. It didn't occur to me that it would be hard to get out of Agnews. I wasn't worried at all about showing the doctors I was normal.

I should have been. Here I was, back at Agnews, a couple of months shy of my eighteenth birthday. It would be more than two years before I was on the street again.

This time around, I was more mature, less fearful. The first time in had been like *One Flew over the Cuckoo's Nest*. Now it was more like *McHale's Navy*.

I had grounds privileges now. There were trees and lawns and benches. As long as you didn't get into trouble, as long as you didn't try to hurt anybody or try to hurt yourself, you could wander around on your own. It was kind of like when I was a kid, when I would go walking along the railroad tracks or take my bike up into the hills.

There was even a bus you could take from the Westside campus, where I was, to the Eastside campus. That's where they kept the *really* crazy people. The bus ride was probably more than a mile, and it felt like being in another world. You could ride that bus and walk around the Eastside and feel like you were in a different city.

I spent a lot of time wandering around at Agnews on my own. Maybe I'd never have gotten into trouble if I'd been alone all the time, but . . .

But you met guys at mealtime. You met guys in the day rooms. Most of them were people you didn't want to know. But I made a couple of friends. I met a guy named Steve Alper.

Steve had been sent to Agnews for some behavior problems. He was skinny and about a foot shorter than me, and he was willing to go along with my schemes, which was very cool. Like always, I needed a partner. I needed a front man. Just like with the great train-station robbery, I always wanted someone around who, if things went wrong, would get caught and then not snitch me off. At Agnews, the second time I was there, that was Steve.

We began to hatch some scams.

The people at Agnews distributed tobacco and rolling papers to anyone who wanted them. But most guys hated the roll-your-owns. They'd pay a lot for real cigarettes. If they didn't have canteen privileges and no one was visiting them and bringing them stuff, they had no way to get real cigarettes. Steve and I had canteen privileges, but we didn't have any real money.

So we cooked up a scam where we could get some money and some real cigarettes in the bargain.

First we'd go to the canteen and buy a pack of cigarettes. We'd open it carefully and take all the cigarettes out. We'd refill the pack with twenty roll-your-owns, and reseal the pack so it looked brand-new. Then we'd sell that pack, as new, to another patient.

If the guy who bought the cigarettes was crazy enough, he didn't notice. If he was just sort of crazy, he might think, *Hey, these cigarettes are a mess.* If he was normal, he might realize something was wrong. So he'd probably take the cigarettes to the canteen and say, "Hey! These are roll-your-owns!" Usually the guy in the canteen would just give him another pack—of real cigarettes.

Sometimes we did that ourselves instead of selling them. It worked so well that after a while we'd just sort of stuff the pack with paper and tobacco. We'd tell the guy at the canteen that there might have been a mistake at the factory.

I thought it was hilarious. It was like these people didn't think we were intelligent enough, or shrewd enough, to figure out any scams. We were in the nuthouse. How smart could we be? So they didn't have any defenses against these little schemes.

There were alcoholics on the ward, and some of them had ways to slip off and buy booze and sneak it back. Some guys drank. Some guys sold liquor. But because it was the 1960s, a lot of people were interested in drugs, too. Some guys sold drugs. Some guys just handed them out. I was given some acid one time. I had what you'd call a bad trip. Later on I took some "orange sunshine" someone gave me, and that was okay.

Since people were interested in drugs, there were ways to make money off them. A friend and I figured out how we could sell marijuana to some of the younger girls at Agnews. Only it wasn't marijuana. Where would guys like us get marijuana? It was just grass cuttings from the lawn. We'd get some of that and dry it out and roll it up in cigarette paper and sell it. We charged one dollar a joint. These girls would come back and tell us what a great trip they had. They wanted more. So me and Steve would string them along. We'd say, "Well, we can get more, but it's going to take a couple of days. And it's going to cost you." Then we'd dry some more grass.

Far more than drugs or alcohol, I was interested in sex. Just like at Rancho Linda, there was plenty of sex at Agnews.

The dormitories were segregated into boys and girls, men and women. The mealtimes were segregated, too. But the classrooms were coed, and so were the grounds. So you could meet girls. You'd see them in class and talk to them afterward. Or you'd see them in the canteen, or sitting on a bench, and you could strike up a conversation.

Getting them alone was a little harder. But it wasn't impossible. Once I was interested in a girl and I knew she was interested in me, I'd go down to the canteen. There was a pay phone there. I'd call the front office and say, "So-and-so has a visitor." Then I'd hang up before they could ask who the visitor was, and I'd head out into the hallway to intercept the girl before she got to the front office. She did have a visitor—me!

To be alone, you'd go for a walk on the grounds. You could take that bus over to the Eastside. Over there the patients were so much crazier that you could do almost anything and no one paid attention.

After a while I figured out which bathrooms were never used. There were some that no one ever went into. That's where I'd take my girls. Usually, because there wasn't much time and there wasn't anyplace to lie down, we wouldn't have actual intercourse. We'd just fool around.

Sometimes I had the real thing, though, like I did with a woman named Ellen. She was older than me, probably in her early thirties, and she was just as into sex as I was. We'd get on the Agnews bus together and go over to the Eastside, where no one knew us by sight. We'd wander around the buildings until we found a place that seemed deserted. We'd have sex in the stairwells. We needed privacy, of course, but we also needed time, because she wore really complicated undergarments—a girdle, and a brassiere that fastened with a million metal hooks—and it took forever to get them off.

I was interested in anyone who was interested in me. This wasn't like with Annette. I would go with anyone who was available and willing. I went with girls my age, and girls who were older. One time I went with this one lady—I don't even want to think about how old she was. Pretty old, though. I'm embarrassed to even remember that.

Daily life at Agnews wasn't difficult. They fed you all right, even if there were rumors about what went into the food. (We heard they put saltpeter in the meals so no one would have any sex drive. They must not have put enough in there for me.) At night you'd watch TV and drink coffee. You got up at five. You went to bed at nine. In between, you played cards a lot. Sometimes no one was around to play with you. I played a lot of solitaire. I played a lot of war—with myself.

After a while, they trusted me enough to give me a job. Part of the deal at Agnews was if you wanted grounds privileges you had to work a job. At first, I cut hair. I guess I wasn't very good at it. By the time I got through with them, everyone had the same haircut. So I didn't last too long at that. Later on, I worked in the bakery, on the hog farm, in the laundry, and in the storerooms. Most of it was boring, stupid work. You didn't really learn anything. You didn't learn enough to get a job on the outside. It was just your way of paying for your keep. If you didn't like it, you could stay confined to your room, which would have been terrible.

There was a lot of hanging out, a lot of time spent just hanging around doing nothing, shooting the breeze. With some of the guys this was okay, and with some of them it wasn't. There was one guy who teased me a lot about sex. He would say I had never had sex with a girl. I'd say that wasn't true, that he was wrong about that. So he'd start asking me questions about it—did I do this, or did I do that? That made me pretty uneasy, so I stayed away from him. I stayed away from anyone who talked about sex. Some guys just gave me the creeps.

But Steve and I got to be friends, and partners. We sold that marijuana together. We did some embezzling, too.

We somehow managed to steal some paperwork from the accounting office, which was the place that banked and disbursed patients' money. I filled out the paperwork. Steve got access to the official stamp. Then he took the paperwork down to the accounting office. When he came back, with his head down and his hands behind him, I thought he'd gotten busted. Then he smiled and showed me his hands. Three hundred dollars!

Another time I cooked up a scheme to sneak out of Agnews. I forged some paperwork requesting that I be allowed to visit my grandmother—Daisy, my mother's mother—in Oakland. I made it look like she had called and made the request. I took the papers in to have them approved. My grandmother didn't actually know anything about it, but I wanted to get out for a few days and have a field trip away from San Jose. I filled out the same kind of paperwork for Steve. We were let out of our wards, and walked to the bus pickup. The Greyhound bus came once a day to the clock tower building. We rode it up to Oakland.

When I was a kid, visiting my grandmother Daisy was a big deal. She still lived in the huge family home on Newton Avenue. It was dark and stately, and felt like money. Sometimes on family visits my uncle Hugh and uncle Gordon were there, and I liked seeing them. But after my father married Lou, we saw my mother's side of the family less and less. My father said bad things about Gordon, and he always felt like Daisy had looked down on him as not good enough for my mother. Maybe seeing them reminded him how much he missed my mother, too. As the years passed, Brian and I were hardly ever taken to see our grandmother anymore.

So when I snuck out of Agnews my grandmother was happy to see me. She had kept up her letter-writing campaign, trying to find out what they were doing to me, and not getting answers that satisfied her. She was relieved to know I was all right. But she seemed surprised that I was able to get to Oakland on my own when I was supposed to be locked up.

Steve and I did that enough times that it turned into an inside joke. When he and I and two other guys formed a little rock band, we called it "Granny's Place." I was the guitar player, Steve played keyboards, another guy played drums, and another guy played bass. We worked up a few songs, like "Louie, Louie," "Wipeout," "Walk, Don't Run," and "House of the Rising Sun." We were good enough that we got to play one of the Agnews dances. They had a real band come in, but when the band took a break we got onstage and did our songs. That was our only gig.

If I'd wanted to, I could have filled out that paperwork and left Agnews for good. But I always came back. Why not? I had nowhere else to go.

Mostly I stayed out of trouble with the staff there, but I did get written up for little things—cutting class, or taking off from work. I never got caught for selling grass, or for going with girls. I never got caught for the embezzling or anything else serious.

But I was a suspect one time in a serious crime that I had nothing to do with. Someone had hot-wired a truck, driven it over to the administration building, broken into the room where they kept the patients' money, stolen the safe where all the money was kept, got the safe onto the truck, and taken it out onto a field. They busted into the safe and made off with a bunch of money.

The administrators thought I was behind this. They brought me in and questioned me. I thought it was a great caper, but—me? How could I do any of that stuff? I didn't know anything about hot-wiring cars, or breaking locks, or cracking safes. And how would I do all of that stuff while I was in my bed, on a locked ward, and still sleeping when they came to talk to me about it? It didn't make sense. Maybe they didn't have any other suspects.

Throughout all this, I had one really good reason not to get in trouble. There was a doctor at Agnews who believed in using electroshock therapy as punishment. Everyone knew about it. I think the technicians *wanted* us to know about it. They wanted us to know what was in store for us if we got out of line.

Steve was one of the people who got out of line. He was friendly with me, but with other people he could be real belligerent. He was a fighter. One day they took Steve out and kept him for a while. A week later, I heard he was out—but they'd moved him to a new ward. They had given him the electroshock.

When I saw him again, he wasn't right. I don't think he was ever right after that. The treatment was supposed to "calm" patients down. In Steve's case, the calm was only temporary. Years later,

Steve would be sent to jail for shooting a wino in the eye with a BB gun after the wino had passed him a bottle of wine that someone had urinated in.

I was afraid of electroshock. I was scared of the medications, too. I had no experience with that, and I was afraid they'd start giving me something that would make me crazy—like the other guys I saw on medication. I didn't know that the doctors had decided not to give me electroshock because I'd had the lobotomy. So my fear of it was very real.

My dad still came to visit me almost every other weekend. He was trying to make up for what happened, I think. He was trying to make it all right.

Other than my dad, my other grandmother, Grandma Boo, was my only visitor at Agnews. She would come once in a while. For some reason she would always come really early in the morning and sleep in her car until visiting hours.

I never saw Lou. I never saw my brothers. When my dad visited, he didn't seem to want to talk about them. He didn't want to talk about me going home. I had given up any ideas about that. I knew they didn't want me there. I knew I couldn't get out of Agnews. I had stopped fantasizing about it, too.

The guy who held the key to me getting out of Agnews was Dr. Shon.

Shon was this balding, bookworm-looking psychiatrist with black-rimmed glasses. He was a nice guy. He dealt with me like it was all a big joke. He'd call me "Mr. Dully," like I was an adult, but it was kind of like he was making fun of me. He'd say, "Well, Mr. Dully, how are you enjoying life here at Agnews?" like he was the owner of a hotel and was asking me whether I was having a good time.

I saw him once a month. He'd ask me questions. Hours and hours of questions. He'd show me inkblots and ask me what I thought of them, or what I saw in them. He never said what he thought about my answers. He'd just nod and ask another question.

After a while, he told me he knew I didn't belong at Agnews. But he also told me I couldn't leave.

I would say, "How can you say that? How can you tell me I don't belong here but I have to stay here anyway?"

He'd smile and say, "That's just the way it is."

The time dragged slowly. It was frustrating to be at Agnews. I didn't know what I could do to make them understand I wasn't crazy, except what I was already doing. And I didn't know how to get out except by showing them I wasn't crazy. But that wasn't working. If Dr. Shon knew I didn't belong there, but told me I couldn't leave, how would I ever get out?

I didn't think of running away, or escaping, because I couldn't imagine where I would go. I didn't think of suicide, either. I was never self-destructive that way. I might have been tired of living, like the song says, but I was also scared of dying. I did not want to die, as lonely or scared or sad as I ever got. I never thought about killing myself.

But it was hard, watching the clock, getting through the days.

Sometime in the middle of 1968—I have no papers on this period of my life, and I wasn't keeping any kind of prison diary at Agnews—Dr. Shon made me an offer. He told me that if I could stay out of trouble for three weeks, he'd arrange to have me released. This meant *no* trouble. I had to go three weeks without screwing up in any way. I couldn't get written up for anything.

That sounded easy. For some guys, it would have been. For me, it was hard. I almost made it, several times. But then I'd get written up for some little infraction or other, ditching a class or not coming down for a meal or something like that.

After a while, Shon decided to let me go anyway. He said, "You're leaving." He didn't say why. He didn't say where. He just said, "We're arranging for your release."

I didn't think I was going home. I didn't think I'd *ever* go home.

I didn't think they could send me back to Juvenile Hall. I was too old. I didn't think they were sending me to prison for the checks, because they told me that was all taken care of.

So I wasn't all that surprised when they said they were sending me back to a halfway house.

I was excited. I had been locked up at Agnews for more than two years. I couldn't wait to get out. I was free again.

At least for a little while.

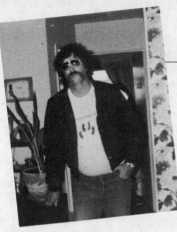

Chapter 12

Homeless

In the spring of 1969, I was moved from Agnews to a halfway house at 884 Jackson Street in Santa Clara, a little white clapboard house not far from Santa Clara University.

It should have been an easy life. I was free. I was taken care of by the government. I got a check every month for $120, which paid my rent and gave me some walking-around money.

But they had rules, and I didn't like following the rules. I was a nonconformist.

Not like the antiwar protestors. I wasn't like them at all. I didn't want to be associated with them.

But I wanted to be associated with *something*. I always did. I knew I wasn't normal. But I wanted to be normal. I wanted to be thought of as normal.

I looked sort of like a biker. I was six feet seven inches, and I weighed about 190 pounds. I had a big bushy mustache. So I started hanging around that Spartan Hub again, drinking with the Gypsy Jokers. Now that I was almost an adult, I could drink more freely. I still didn't like it all that much. I didn't like the taste. But I liked the buzz. I liked Budweiser. I liked the girlie drinks, too. I started drinking sloe gin fizz. That was my drink.

I wasn't a difficult drunk. I didn't get in fights. I didn't have hangovers. I didn't do wild things. I was kind of a happy drunk.

But my drinking might have gotten in the way of my residence at the halfway house. They had these rules, like curfew. You had to be in by a certain time of night. You had to do things their way, or you were out. So they asked me to leave.

I had recently met a guy named Dave Sawyer. I was walking down the street. He was driving along in a white Chevy with red flames painted on the side. He pulled over and asked me if I wanted to cruise around. I didn't have anything better to do, so I said yes. We started hanging around together a little.

When I got kicked out of the halfway house, Sawyer and his girlfriend, Lynn, invited me to move into their place on Third Street in San Jose.

It was a studio apartment, which meant there was one big room attached to a little kitchen. There was one bed. It was a big bed, but it was just one bed. There was no hanky-panky, but that's how we slept.

Lynn was on welfare. We used her welfare check to pay the rent. I was on government relief—ATD, which meant Aid to the Totally Disabled, or something like that. My check paid for everything else. We used my money to eat and party on.

Dave and I would take the Chevy cruising, looking for something to do. We'd go pick up girls. We'd go hang out in a restaurant. We'd go drink someplace. It was kind of a dumb way to live. I had nothing to do, and no reason to do it. I had no work ethic, and I never looked for work. I didn't really have to. The government check came every month. All I had to do was be the guy who had the lobotomy.

But I couldn't just go along and not do *something*. So I started doing something bad, again. I started writing bad checks again.

It wasn't some big criminal enterprise. It was just writing checks against funds that weren't there. I'd open a bank account with a little money, and then start writing checks for larger and larger amounts. Like before, I'd use a check to buy something from a pawnshop, then I'd take it to a different pawnshop and turn it into money. It was an easy way to get some money fast.

It was also an easy way to get caught, and I got caught. Lynn and I had gone into this bank that was across the street from some city government offices. They didn't know me in that bank. They didn't know I didn't have any money in my account. I knew I could write a check and get some cash.

But there was a customer in the bank who worked for the police department—in the fraud unit. She recognized me from my mug shot. She tipped the bank off, and someone got the cops over there, and we were arrested before we even left the building.

It was a Tuesday. They held me overnight, I think, and let me go on my own recognizance the following morning. I hadn't even bothered to call my dad to see about getting bail. Those days were gone.

I had already spent quite a few nights in jail. One more night didn't rehabilitate me. By Friday morning of that same week, I was in trouble again.

Sawyer and I had been riding around that day in the Chevy. We had guns—a pair of pistols. We had bought them with a bad check at a pawnshop. I'm not sure what we were going to do with them. We weren't going to rob anybody with them, or hurt anybody, because I was not into anything like that. We weren't going to rob a bank. I think we had them because when we went into a pawnshop with a bad check, we had to buy something, and there was nothing else in that pawnshop we wanted.

When a police car came up behind us that Friday morning, I threw my gun out the window. Dave stashed his in the glove compartment.

That was stupid. The cops pulled us over. They had a look in the glove compartment. They found the gun. Then they looked in the trunk. They found some tools. It was probably just pliers and stuff. But to these cops, they looked like burglary tools. So they arrested us on a bunch of charges, including robbery, burglary, receiving stolen property, and possession of burglary tools.

Since it was a Friday, I got to spend the weekend in jail. I was released on Monday morning. The charges were all dismissed.

They let me off, and what got me off again was the lobotomy.

Judges probably don't want to take advantage of the disadvantaged, and it was obvious that I had real disadvantages. The operation put me at a real disadvantage.

I personally think the real disadvantage was that no one ever taught me how to *do* anything. I was almost twenty-one, and I had no idea how to take care of myself. So, in a way, I used that disadvantage to my own advantage, by playing on it when I was in trouble to get out of trouble.

It worked. My arrest record shows one run-in after another. It also shows what a smart-ass I was. I'm listed as having at least seven criminal aliases—like I was some kind of big-time crook. I had told the police that I was Vion Vaccura, Paul Weston, Vion Dully, Vion Dulley, Vion Richard Dix, Richard Dicks, and Kirk Lee Dix.

Where did I come up with this stuff? I don't even remember half of those phony names. I remember that Vion Vaccura was a stage name I made up for myself back when I thought I was going to be a rock star. Paul Weston was a guy I knew from school. Kirk Lee was my baby brother's name. But Richard Dicks, or Dix? I can only imagine that, since my stepbrother George's last name was Cox, I was making some sort of stupid pun out of Cox and Dix.

Whatever it was, it didn't turn the authorities against me. The judge let me off. He let Sawyer off, too. I guess there hadn't been any bank robberies they could blame us for. They let us both go.

For Dave, it didn't last long. He had met a girl who had been at Agnews. She was young and cute and he liked her, and they started going around together. Dave and I were still living with Lynn, and Dave was with Lynn, and this girl wanted Dave to leave Lynn and come be with her. Dave didn't want to.

So, the girl turned him over to the cops. See, she was only fourteen or fifteen years old. She looked about twenty-three, but she was a minor. And they had been sleeping together. She told the cops. They came looking for Dave. He got convicted of statutory rape, and he went to jail.

I stayed on living with Lynn in that studio apartment on Third Street. We were fooling around now, but it wasn't anything serious.

Besides, not long after that I met Martha.

Martha was a big girl with a round face and dark skin and dark hair that she wore in a little page-boy style. She had also been a patient at Agnews. Her whole name was Martha Bishop. Her father was Cecil Bishop and her mother's sister was a Lankershim. I didn't know the whole family story, but I knew the Bishop name was famous, and I knew that the Lankershim family owned a bunch of the San Fernando Valley down in Los Angeles. I knew there was money in that family.

One day me and my old friend Ed Woodson, who I knew from my first halfway house, were riding around in this limousine. I'm not sure exactly what we thought we were doing in the limousine, but we had rented it using a bad check, of course, and we were just cruising around.

Ed saw Martha and told the driver to pull over. We got into a conversation with her. She saw that we had a bucket of fried chicken in the limo, and she was hungry. We told her we needed some money to pay for the limo, and she had some money. So we made a deal: our chicken, her money. She got in and started eating fried chicken.

I took her back to my place, and she never left.

My father had always told me to stay away from the women at Agnews. He said, "Whatever you do, don't get involved with anyone from that place." So going with Martha was a way of telling my dad that he couldn't tell me what to do. I also liked Martha for the sex.

We drank a lot. We danced a lot. Martha moved into the little studio apartment with me and Lynn, and we set up house. We'd go out, and have these wild nights. After about a year and a half, we decided to make it official. We got married at a Lutheran church in Mountain View. I invited my dad to the wedding, but he didn't come. Martha's mom came, but her dad refused, too. My uncle Orville and aunt Evelyn came. Martha's brother was there. It was a small wedding. Afterward, we went to this restaurant in Palo Alto for the reception.

We had such big dreams and ambitions. We were married! We were going to make it together! We were going to live the good life!

But we didn't have the first idea how. We weren't working. We didn't have jobs. We didn't know how to get jobs. We both had this checkered past. And we had a way to get along that didn't require working. I got a government check. So did she. Plus her parents gave her money. So we never had jobs or had to get them.

After a while we got our own place. Then Martha came into some money from her aunt. Her parents were worried that I'd get all the money, so they used it to buy her a condominium.

Now we were property owners. The condominium was on Bouret Drive. It had white walls and Chinese red carpets. We moved in and that was supposed to be our life.

But we didn't have a life. We didn't have a real marriage. We had a kind of association. We were just playing at marriage. I wanted to have my cake and eat it, too, which meant I wanted to be with Martha, but I wanted to be with any other woman I could get my hands on. And Martha wanted to be with everybody.

We stayed together from 1970 to 1975.

It was not a good time. We got into drugs. We were smoking a lot of marijuana, and doing a drug we called "KJ," which was a kind of tranquilizer. We were doing "rocket fuel," which was like angel dust sprinkled on marijuana. I was taking a lot of Dexedrine, too. I had found some outside a doctor's office, and started taking it. I liked it, so I just kept taking it.

It was a weird way to live. We had a very drunken, druggy life. We had terrible fights. I became violent, too, which was unusual for me. Maybe it was the marriage, maybe it was the drugs, or maybe it was both, but it was *bad*.

We had bought a boat, a little sailboat. It cost eight hundred dollars, and I was paying it off a little at a time, and we'd go sailing out of Santa Cruz. We didn't really know how to sail, but we'd take the boat out and pretend. One time she did something stupid and almost knocked me overboard. I got so mad that I actually hit her.

I hadn't ever hit a woman before. I had practically never hit a man, since I was a kid. It was shocking, even to me.

Martha got even by having me arrested—not for that, but for other things. She'd get mad at me and she'd call the police and snitch me off, for things like parking tickets and warrants for traffic tickets.

This happened more than a couple of times. I spent a lot of time in the Santa Clara County Jail. Usually it was just overnight, or for a few days at a time, but I got to know it pretty well. It held between three hundred and five hundred men. They were segregated into sections, and the sections all had names. There was "Max Row," which was maximum security. There was "Siberia," because it was cold all the time. There was "Hollywood," and "Snake Pit," but I don't know why they were called that. There was "Queen's Row," and everybody knew what that was all about.

I had been in Max Row for the bad checks. Now I was mostly in Hollywood. It wasn't so bad, and it wasn't for long.

My dad would usually find out I was being arrested, sometimes before the cops showed up. He had continued to do part-time work in law enforcement, so he knew a lot of the police officers. They'd get a warrant to pick me up, and they'd look at my paperwork. They'd see a guy who was really big and who had a lot of arrests. They'd call my dad and say, "We gotta pick him up. Are we gonna have a problem?" My dad would say, "No. He's a pussycat."

It was true. I never resisted. I never gave the cops a hard time. I wasn't violent with them. I had no capacity for it. I couldn't really fight. I had studied karate for a short time, with a guy I knew who was an instructor. I got up to blue belt, but then I broke my toe doing a leg sweep. That hurt! I didn't know karate was supposed to hurt. So I never went back.

Sometimes my dad would come and post bail. Usually he wouldn't. One time around 1972, I got arrested for outstanding warrants for unpaid parking tickets and moving violations. I was twenty-three or twenty-four. I knew the bail was about $1,200. My dad came to visit me. He took out his wallet, and he spread out this fan of money—a lot of money. He said, "I've got the bail money, right here. I could go in there and bail you out. But I'm not going to. I'm going to let you stay in here awhile."

My dad *never* carried around that kind of money. There was no reason in the world he would have that kind of money on him except to show it to me.

So that meant he had found out how much the bail was, then he had gone to the bank, withdrawn the money, and come down to the jail to show me the $1,200—just so he could say he wasn't going to use it to post my bail. He did all that to teach me a lesson.

I guess I didn't learn the lesson.

The next time I got arrested was in Fernley, Nevada, a town to the northeast of Reno. I was up there with Martha and my old pal Dave Sawyer, who had already done his time for being with the underage girl and gotten out. I don't know what we were doing in that part of Nevada. We had no business in Fernley. But it was nighttime, and we were tired, so we decided to sleep in the car.

I was in the driver's seat when the cops rolled up, and the key was in the ignition. I was carrying a suspended driver's license. So they hauled me in. They let Martha and Dave go.

The judge said one week in jail or $110. Well, if I'd had $110 I wouldn't have been sleeping in the car. So I took the week.

Martha and Dave took the car and left, probably for San Jose. What else were they going to do? They didn't have any money, either. So it's not like they could just rent a room and hang around and wait for me to get out.

I got out a week later. I was alone, and I was a good long way from home. I had a little money in my pocket, but not much. It was enough for me to get either a good meal or a Greyhound ticket back to San Jose.

But I wanted both. I wanted to go home, but I was hungry, and I wanted a good meal. So I did the only intelligent thing I could think of. I took my money into a casino and gambled it. I figured I could turn it into enough money for the bus ticket and the good meal.

I lost the money. I had to hitchhike back to San Jose on an empty stomach.

It was pretty low. But I was used to living pretty low. I had lived on a $120-a-month government check with a wife. When you've been at the bottom, nothing looks that bad, and I had been at the bottom for quite a while. The bottom was *normal* for me.

But the bottom got worse.

Freeman had stopped paying attention to me some years before. I don't know what the circumstance was—did I see him, or did he receive a visit from Lou?—but he made some final notes in late 1969:

> *Howard has been out of Agnews for the past year and is making a very unsatisfactory adjustment. He has been in jail on several occasions, and is at present on probation.*
>
> *He is conspicuous with his long hair, dirty clothes, and he associates mostly with co-patients of Agnews, and he claims to have married a girl although he is so untruthful generally that it's hard to believe that any girl would accept him. He sponges on his friends, borrows money from friends of the family. Nobody seems to be able to get through to him, the psychiatric technicians, the parole officers and other officers.*

Freeman was having a bad time, too. His marriage had not improved with the move to California, and neither had his wife's health. She developed into a full-blown alcoholic. She'd spend the whole day drinking while Freeman was out seeing patients. Freeman had to ask liquor stores in the neighborhood not to sell her booze.

Two of Freeman's adult children were living in the Bay Area, and he saw them often. Another of his children, though, had met a tragic end, in Freeman's beloved Yosemite.

One summer, Freeman had taken two of his boys for their annual camping trip. They were hiking near the top of Vernal Falls on a hot summer morning when Freeman's second youngest boy discovered that his canteen was empty. Freeman had forgotten to remind him to fill it. Freeman pointed at the nearby Merced River, and told him to fill it there.

The boy slipped into the river and began to float downstream, toward the falls. Another hiker, a sailor on shore leave, saw the boy and jumped in to save him. While Freeman and his other son watched, the boy and the sailor went over the falls together— falling 325 feet to the rocks below. It was months before the boy's body was recovered. Freeman's wife, traveling in the East, read about her son's death in a local newspaper.

Freeman buried himself in work. He continued to believe in the lobotomy, and wrote long papers on its usefulness, despite the fact that new drugs had come along that did a better job, had fewer side effects, and were not irreversible.

One of the papers was called "Adolescents in Distress" and bragged about the "therapeutic possibilities of lobotomy" on children.

He started by observing that a lot of teenagers are anxious, but said this was healthy. "A certain amount of anxiety is good for a boy or a girl, in the same way that a certain amount of fleas is good for a dog—keeps him from thinking about being a dog."

Freeman reported several case studies of young people he had given lobotomies to over the years.

One was a boy identified as R.W. He began having problems at fourteen, hearing voices and thinking God and the devil were after him, and became convinced that he was going to die. Freeman gave him a lobotomy in 1958 at Herrick Memorial Hospital in Berkeley. Five years later, he could not care for himself, even though his hallucinations had never returned.

Another patient of Freeman's, identified as Carol, was also lobotomized at Herrick around the same time. Her mother was a schizophrenic living at Agnews. Carol suffered from horrible anxiety. Freeman treated her with "intensive" electroshock treatment. When that didn't produce the desired results, Freeman gave her a lobotomy. A few months later, Freeman could report that Carol was living with her grandmother, helping with the housework, doing well in school, popular with the boys, and not subject to fits of anxiety. Freeman wrote, "The girl's personality has undoubtedly been changed by lobotomy. Once the anxiety was relieved a lively and friendly personality emerged."

A third patient, A.W., had been in very bad shape before her surgery, also at Herrick, and was in pretty bad shape afterward, too. It wasn't clear whether she had benefited in any way from the lobotomy.

The fourth patient was identified as R.C. Like me, he had received his lobotomy in 1960 at Doctors General Hospital in San Jose. Prior to his surgery he had been housed for several years at the Langley Porter Clinic, and later at Agnews, where he had spent most of his time in bed. He was hostile and had feelings of sensitivity and inadequacy. After a series of forty electroshock treatments brought him only "fleeting" relief, Freeman performed the lobotomy. He was able to report, with real enthusiasm, that R.C. returned home right after the surgery, became more cheerful and alert, and got along better with his older brother. "His feelings were less easily hurt, and he seemed less self-conscious. He is now in a period of rehabilitation at Goodwill Industries. Thus within a year the young man has made more progress socially than in the preceding ten."

This guy almost sounds like me. Trouble at home, trouble with his brother, and after surgery stuck in a go-nowhere job with Goodwill.

But he's not me. The R.C. in this paper, and the A.W., are Richard and Ann, the kids who drove with me to Freeman's disastrous meeting at Langley Porter Clinic when we were all booed off the stage.

Freeman doesn't mention that in his report. In fact, he cheats a little. He says in his report that Richard suffered from "helplessness," characterized by his typical comment on everything: "I'm doing the best I can." But he suggests this was a problem *before* the surgery. In fact, that's what Richard kept saying on the stage that day at Langley. That's what freaked those doctors out.

Freeman's career wasn't going well at all. The embarrassment at Langley Porter, he later said, had a serious effect on his reputation. Added to it, Freeman had attempted to do to another child what he had done to me, and he had gotten in trouble for it.

On May 31, 1961, five months after the trip to the clinic, he wrote to several of his old colleagues, including James Watt, the surgeon who had assisted him in all his early lobotomies, asking for support.

> *Dear Jim,*
>
> *I am being savagely attacked by the Chief of Pediatrics at the Palo Alto–Stanford hospital for even recommending a lobotomy in a 12-year-old boy who, according to my lights, is going to end up in an institution. This pediatrician has convinced the executive committee of the medical staff of Palo Alto that I should be denied renewal of membership on the staff. That seems to put me in the class of the abortionists and the rapists, the drug users, etc. I would appreciate it if you would write to [him] indicating that lobotomy is a recognized method of treatment of emotionally disturbed children, and not a heinous offense.*

Several of his old associates wrote letters in his defense, but the campaign was not successful. Freeman's membership to the hospital was not renewed. A couple of years later, he was also asked to leave El Camino Hospital—which he personally had helped build—because of his use of electroshock on a woman who had been found wandering the streets. She was brought to El Camino by the police, and was incoherent. Freeman administered an "emergency" electroshock, without conducting a proper examination, or getting permission from her family, or taking head X-rays, or observing the hospital's traditional two-day waiting period.

Then, in 1967, Freeman made his last medical mistake. He had agreed to perform a lobotomy on a woman he had first met in 1946. She was among his first lobotomy patients. The operation was a success, but she had suffered some relapses. Freeman conducted a second lobotomy in 1956. Now she was back for a third.

This time it didn't go well. Freeman had her admitted to Herrick. During the surgery he ripped a blood vessel in her brain. She began to bleed. She died a few hours after the surgery.

Freeman was seventy-two. That was his final lobotomy.

But it wasn't his final word on the procedure. Freeman had continued to communicate with his former patients—remember those Christmas cards?—and he now began touring the country, visiting with them, examining them, comparing their lives now to their lives before the lobotomies. He logged thousands of miles in a specially equipped camper van, another version of his famous Lobotomobile. It's like he was looking as hard as he could for evidence that his surgery was as useful as he always insisted it was, and that the patients who didn't get better were the exception instead of the rule.

His health was failing. Freeman had been treated for cancer several times in the 1960s, always bouncing back and returning at once to work. After his wife died, he continued to live alone in the San Jose area. He continued to hike in the Sierras, returning often to Yosemite.

He may have suffered from depression, or anxiety, himself. He once told an interviewer that he had taken a dose of nembutol, which is a very powerful and highly addictive barbiturate, to help him sleep—every single night for more than thirty years. He didn't consider himself an addict, he said, because he had "rarely" needed more than three capsules a night. He said, "I have found it most helpful."

In 1972, Freeman's cancer returned. He was hospitalized in San

Francisco in May. He fell into a coma and died in the hospital, with his children at his side, a month later.

Martha and I had broken up. I don't know where she went. I wound up living in a dirt lot.

I had hooked up again with Ed Woodson. He was working as a night watchman at a used-car lot down on Stockton Avenue, near the old Del Monte canning factory. Between shifts he lived in an empty lot by the railroad yard.

It was a big clear lot, shaded by a huge pepper tree, about twenty feet from the street and about thirty feet from the railroad tracks. A few abandoned cars were scattered around. There was a bunch of us who lived there, sleeping outside.

At first, it was fun. It was like being cowboys. You slept outside on the dirt in blankets. When it rained, you'd grab a blanket and climb into one of the abandoned cars. It was cozy. There was an old Corvair that I could sleep in. If it rained, or if I was with a girl, I'd spend the night in there.

We spent our time drinking or finding money to drink with. You'd spent part of the day looking for food, part of the day trying to get cleaned up, part of the day trying to get money for booze, and the rest of the day and night drinking.

If you had a little money, you could buy a shower at a place called Truckadero on First Street. It was a truck stop and they sold showers there. If you were hungry, there was an A&W root beer place across the street. You could get a hot dog there real cheap. I ate a lot of hot dogs. If you wanted to drink in a bar, there was a place called Pedro's just up the block. I spent a lot of nights in Pedro's boozing it up.

Getting money for booze was like our job. We'd find stuff to sell, and we'd steal it. We'd take these huge metal plates from the old Del Monte cannery and haul them over to a scrap-metal yard and sell them for money.

Those were hard days.

Somewhere in there I met a girl who was hanging around with Dave Sawyer. Her name was Laurie. Dave had always been trying to get my girls away from me. This time I got his girl away from him. She had a little apartment in University Square, over by Santa Clara University. I moved in. We lived off my welfare money, which wasn't really enough to pay the rent and keep the lights and telephone on and buy food. So, I quit drinking to save money.

We lived that way for more than a year, then she left me—for a girl. Not long after, I found myself in another place, living with a girl named Claire. That lasted a few weeks. Then I was back on the lot with Sawyer and the other guys. I went back to hanging out in Pedro's.

One of the regulars was a girl named Christine Heriman. One night in 1977 she invited me to join her and a friend. We had a few beers, then went across the street to another bar. Christine started feeding me Black Russians. By the time Christine invited me to come home with her, I was so drunk I couldn't remember who I was supposed to be with—her or her friend. She said I was with her.

Christine was a dark-eyed, curly-haired woman with a big smile. She was big all over. I liked that. I liked girls who looked like they ate regular. She looked like she ate plenty. When we got to her house, I took a look in her refrigerator. There was a plate of pork chops. I took one look at those pork chops and said, "Howard's not going to go hungry for a while."

Love has to start somewhere. For me, it started with the pork chops.

But the next morning I had a kind of rude awakening. I got up to use the restroom. I saw baby furniture in the spare bedroom. She had a kid? Later that day, I met the kid. He was a cute toddler named Justin. Christine told me that his father had split. He and Christine had never gotten married.

That was good enough for me. I moved in.

Christine was pretty good at taking care of herself. She wasn't shy about asking for help. She was good at borrowing stuff and not giving it back—stuff like cash. She had a special way of getting people to help her and then not care if she never returned the favor, or the money. That's how we lived.

Christine and I had our issues right from the start. She was a lot like Lou. She was headstrong and willful, and she didn't have a lot of compassion. But I used her as my even keel.

For a while we managed these apartments called the Rock Springs, on Rock Spring Drive. We lived in the front unit, and we took care of the other units.

But it was like living in Peyton Place. Chris decided things weren't working out with us. She moved out. That same day, I moved in with a girl named Janice who lived across the street. Then Chris ran off to Lake Tahoe with a guy who lived in one of the Rock Springs units. They got married. But two weeks later, Chris was back in town. She wanted me to move back in. I moved back in. The man she had married, it turned out, was gay. The marriage was never consummated, and it lasted only two weeks.

Then Chris decided we had to get out of town, to get away from all the people we knew, so we could start to live better. We moved to Bend, Oregon. We were going to change cities and change our lives.

It didn't last long. Six months later, we were back. We moved in with Chris's sister Cindy and her husband, Henry, on the east side of San Jose. Henry was an ex-con. He and Cindy had one son. Cindy had a son from another relationship. Henry didn't work. I wasn't working. Chris wasn't working. Cindy was a dispatcher for an ambulance company. Somehow the four of us, with the three little kids, lived in a two-bedroom house.

Then we had to get our own place. Chris was pregnant. I was the father.

This was a big surprise to me. I had been told, since Agnews, that I couldn't have children, that I would never have children. Maybe they told me that because they thought I *shouldn't* have children, but that's not the way I heard it. If I was with a girl, I never took any precaution, and all through the years I had never gotten anyone pregnant—as far as I knew.

Then Christine got pregnant, and in 1979 we had a son. I named him Rodney, after my father. He would be Rodney Lester Dully—the Lester was for Chris's father—instead of Rodney Lloyd Dully.

I don't remember my family being around much then. My father didn't visit when Rodney was born. But I did have a visit from my stepbrother George. He was down from Washington, visiting with my dad, and he wanted to get together.

I was nervous about seeing him. It had been years since we'd met, and we hadn't spent any real time together since before my lobotomy. I was afraid I'd say the wrong thing, or we'd start talking about the past and I'd say something to make him mad.

He was really nervous about the meeting, too—but for different reasons. He was afraid of me. Lou had convinced him that I was dangerous, that he and his family wouldn't be safe having me around. Lou had said I was "predatory and scary," he said, "a paranoid schizophrenic and unpredictable." George told me Lou had started using those exact words right after I had my operation, and had continued using them for years afterward.

I learned later that Lou had told Brian the same things, and also made him think I was dangerous and not to be trusted.

Brian had finished high school and gone on to college, at UC Davis. But he was still living at home, until something happened with Lou and my dad. Things between them were very distant. They didn't seem to want to be married to each other anymore. They argued frequently.

One day Lou took Brian aside. She was worried about Rod, she said. She was afraid he was becoming violent. She was afraid he would try to hurt her, or hurt Brian. So she gave him some advice: If your father gets violent with you, she said, "You should get a hammer and sneak up behind him and hit him hard right on the back of the head. That will kill him."

Despite Lou's warnings the meeting with George went fine. We had coffee. We talked. I was surprised by what he talked about. He *wanted* to talk about the old days, and about what happened to me. He felt guilty about it. He told me he knew I had been mistreated when we were boys. He felt like my lobotomy and my years at Agnews and Rancho Linda were somehow *his* fault.

I said, "George! You were twelve years old! What could you do?"

He said something about how he should have stood up for me.

I said, "How? Were you supposed to get in trouble just because I was getting in trouble? It wouldn't have made any difference."

He didn't look convinced. He still looked scared, and like he felt guilty. It would be more than twenty years before I saw him again.

Now that I was a dad, I had to start becoming responsible. Chris and I moved with the boys into our own place, and I got a job working for a company that managed mobile-home parks. I did maintenance on swimming pools and hot tubs. I did some gardening. I was in charge of reading the gas meters.

I liked the work, but I liked the stuff that happened after work better. There was a woman who cut hair in one of the mobile-home parks. I went in one night after hours and asked her to cut my hair. She did, and some things happened. Nice things. And those nice things continued to happen.

Christine knew something was going on. She knew I was seeing someone. But she couldn't figure out who. So she started tailing me when I left the house.

One night she saw me and the hairdresser leaving the mobile-home park, and followed us. But somehow she followed the wrong car. She ended up going into this bar where she thought she'd find us. When we weren't there, she went back outside to the car she'd been following and slashed the tires—of some other person's car.

I was already out of town. The hairdresser had a friend in Visalia. We had decided to go down there and visit.

By the time I got back to San Jose, Christine was mad. I called her at home, from some bar, and said I was on my way. She said she didn't want me coming home. She was upset. She wanted to talk first. So when she told me to meet her in this shopping center parking lot, I agreed.

I was standing beside my car when she showed up. It was dark. It was late. There was no one around. She drove into the parking lot and over to where I was standing—fast. I realized almost too late that she was going to run me down. I dove and rolled out of the way just in time.

She was jealous like that. Another time she was going through my wallet and found a picture of a naked girl I was trying to set up with a friend of mine. Chris didn't want an explanation. She came at me with a steak knife.

We always patched things up. But Chris's jealousy meant I had to stay away from the woman in the picture, and I had to quit the mobile-home-management job.

I needed another job. So I got one, helping out in a print shop. I got good enough at printing that when the boss decided to sell the business, I borrowed four thousand dollars from my dad and set up shop.

For a while, things were good. I was living the high life. I hung out in a bar called The Golden Horn. I'd go in there with a pocket full of money. I'd start drinking Black Russians, and ordering drinks for all the girls. I'd wind up dancing, and end up going home with girls I hardly even knew. I'd go through $500 just like that.

So I lost the printing business. I couldn't cover our overhead. I tried. I had even stopped paying the rent on our house as a way of keeping the business going. When we got evicted from that house, we moved into the print shop. I thought that would be a good way to cut down expenses. Imagine, two adults and two little boys living in a print shop in the middle of downtown San Jose. This was my idea of how to save money. It didn't work. I lost the shop.

With no money, and no place to live, Chris and I had to move in with Nancy, another sister. But Nancy didn't like my drinking. She wouldn't let me sleep in the house. So I spent most nights sleeping in this old GMC truck my dad had given me.

It wasn't just the business I was messing up. It was my marriage, too. I was chasing a woman who lived in South San Jose. She wasn't that interested in me, but she was very interested in cocaine. I'd go visit her and bring some coke along. She'd do the coke. I'd drink. She'd do some more coke. I'd drink some more, and wait for her to decide to have sex with me. I figured that sooner or later she would get high enough to let me sleep with her, but she never did.

I always had a lot to drink before I went home. One night, I had too much. By the time I left her house, I was drunk and sleepy. So I decided to take a little nap.

Unfortunately I was still driving at the time. I went to sleep and the truck kept going. It plowed into the side of a parked van.

The impact woke me up. I knew I would be taken to jail if they caught me. I had no money to pay for the van I'd just smashed into. So I drove home.

It didn't occur to me that I had a drinking problem, but I knew I had a life problem. I knew I wasn't happy. While all this craziness was going on, I was trying to do something about that. It just took me a while to get past the craziness and into something more normal.

It took Barbara.

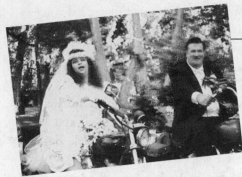

Barbara

$\int$ he likes to joke it was love at first sight—on her part. She and Christine were friends working together at a convalescent hospital called Our Lady of Fatima Villa. Christine was the cook. Barbara was the dishwasher. They had started hanging around together. Barbara says the first time she saw me, I was passed out on the couch, lying on my side, snoring. She thought I looked like a ruffian. She was impressed by my size, and when I woke up she liked the sound of my voice. She said, half-joking, "That's the man for me."

I liked her, too. But at that time I liked all the girls. I was interested in Limey Lou, and Roxanne, and Lana, and Tammy, and some other girls whose names I don't remember—or maybe I didn't even know their names back then. I had a roving eye.

At first, Barbara was just Chris's friend from work. Then she started babysitting for us, spending the evening with Justin and Rodney while Chris and I went out.

She was great. She was cute, and she was smart, and she was funny. She was originally from Chicago. Her dad worked for the San Jose *Mercury*. Her mom, who worked for the *Los Gatos Weekly-Times,* had been a dancer in New York. She once dated Marlon Brando.

Barbara was the youngest of five kids. She was the last one

living at home when her mom and dad decided to get a divorce— and when her mom, right after that, was diagnosed with terminal brain cancer. The doctors gave her a few months to live. Her dad decided not to go through with the divorce. Barbara was only fifteen when her mother died.

She had been sick a lot while Barbara was growing up. She was very overweight, and she had diabetes, and glaucoma, and heart disease. When she got the brain cancer, and got really sick, Barbara hated the way the nurses treated her.

That's how she got interested in health care. She knew there was a better way to treat people who were seriously ill. When she was sixteen she went to work for Our Lady of Fatima Villa, where she met Chris. By the time I met her, she was good enough friends with Chris that she knew something I didn't know: Chris was fooling around behind my back. She had a boyfriend at work, a dishwasher named Brian. So Barbara probably wasn't all that surprised when I started showing an interest in her.

My relationship with Chris was bad. Our life together was bad. But our boys needed a proper home. So when the opportunity came for us to move to our own house, we grabbed it—even if the arrangement was a little unconventional. Chris and I had terrible credit ratings, and we didn't have a lot of cash on hand. But Barbara had a great credit rating, and she had some money saved up. So we decided to combine forces and move in together. Barbara's name went on the lease, and her money paid the security deposit.

Barbara had already put down another security deposit—on *me*. Christine had borrowed two thousand dollars and never paid it back. Barbara likes to joke that she purchased me for two thousand dollars. She says, "I had to *buy* you to get you."

Barbara could see that Chris and I were breaking up. She wanted to be with me, but she did not want to bust up my relationship with my kids. She did not want to be the reason why I stopped being a good father.

So we all moved into the Kelley Park Garden Apartments, on Owsley Avenue. It was in a bad neighborhood. The police arrested a man for shooting up in our carport the day we moved in. There were always people hanging out in front of our building, drinking beer and playing their music too loud. It was a terrible place to raise kids.

But I wasn't a bad dad. For a lot of my kids' childhood, I was a stay-at-home parent. Christine worked full-time. Barb worked full-time. I had mostly part-time jobs, and so I was the one at home most of the time.

I was no Mr. Mom. First, I wasn't any good at diapers. It wasn't that I didn't like it. I just couldn't do it. I don't know why. I could rebuild an engine, but I could never make the diapers stay on. I tried everything, from a staple gun to duct tape. They wouldn't stay on.

I was always afraid I was using the wrong powder or ointment, too, and I was afraid to hold the boys when they were babies. They were so little. They seemed like tiny pieces of breakable china. I was so afraid of hurting them. I couldn't wait until they got older and I could play with them.

Then they started to grow up, and that's when I became a really good parent. I did yard duty when the kids were in elementary school. I went out and bought flag football equipment for them, because the school didn't have any of that stuff. I did Little League with my boys. I even stayed at the elementary school with the flag football teams for several years after my kids left that school.

But I wasn't much of a mate. I had become an abusive drunk. I liked to yell, and I liked to argue. I'd come home drunk some nights and wake Chris up just so I could yell at her. "What do you mean you're asleep? Wake up and fight!" I was impossible.

One night I got so mad that I hit her. It was the second time in my life I had hit a woman, and it filled me with shame. To make things worse, I wasn't working during this period. I hadn't been working steady for a long time. I'd get a little job, or I'd start a little business, but it was always a crummy job or a business that went nowhere.

For example, before the print shop failed, I started rebuilding car engines in my garage. When I ran out of room in the garage, I moved the business into the house. I rebuilt a Porsche engine right in my living room.

Later, I worked at McDonald's. I was the guy who did the stuff no one else wanted to do. I unloaded the truck. I cleaned the fry vats and the flues. I tried cooking for a while, but they told me I was going to be the guy who cleaned the vats. They told me that was a *promotion.*

For a while I was a gardener. But I didn't enjoy the work, and I never got the knack of estimating the jobs right.

After that, I had a job driving a tow truck, working as a repo man. I knew a guy who had a Ford pickup with a hydraulic lift on it. He did repossessions for a pot lot—one of those used-car lots with the signs in front that say WE FINANCE and EZ CREDIT. People would fall behind in their payments, and the pot lot owner would call us and we'd go get the car. He'd pay $125 or $150 per car.

I don't remember why I stopped doing the repo work. But pretty soon I wasn't working again.

That meant I had more time for drinking and hanging around. My favorite place during those days was The Saddle Rack, this big cowboy bar down in San Jose. One day in mid-1985 I was in there drinking rum and Cokes.

Barbara was at work, and I had her car—a nice yellow Capri, which in those days was a pretty hot little car. It was in the repair shop. I was supposed to pick it up when it was done and then go pick Barbara up at work.

But I was drunk. So of course I got to the shop late and picked up the car late and got to Barbara's work late. She had already gotten a ride home from someone else. So I started driving home.

Because I was drunk I ran out of gas on the freeway. I grabbed a gas can from the trunk and started walking toward this gas station I could see off in the distance.

A California Highway Patrol officer stopped and asked what the trouble was. I showed him the gas can. He offered to drive me down to the station.

I got in the car. I knew I smelled like alcohol. I thought honesty might be the best policy. So I said to him, "I been drinking a little."

He said, "You look okay to me."

The CHP officer dropped me at the gas station and took off. I bought the gas and carried the can back up the freeway. I was just pulling away when the same CHP officer reappeared in my rearview mirror. He pulled me over and arrested me for DUI. I was hauled in and booked and fingerprinted.

One more time, it was my dad who came down and posted my bail.

It was late when he drove me home. Chris was sitting on the sofa with Brian—the dishwasher she was having her affair with.

I blew up. I started yelling. I shouted at Brian, "What the hell are you doing here?" I shouted at Chris, "What the hell is going on here?" Brian took off, fast. Chris didn't have any answers that I liked. So I told her, "I'm leaving. I want you out of here when I get back."

When I came home, it was three o'clock in the morning and Chris and the boys were gone. Chris moved into an apartment on Alum Rock Avenue, taking Justin and Rodney with her. Barbara and I stayed in the house.

But I wasn't done with Chris. I was angry when I found out she had been cheating on me with Brian—even though I had been doing the same thing with Barbara. So I began to fight for custody of Rodney.

To be honest, I wasn't interested in his welfare. I was only interested in hurting Chris. I didn't realize that separating Rodney from

Justin was cruel. So was demanding custody of Rodney and leaving Justin behind. His real father had abandoned him. Now I was abandoning him, too.

But I won. I got Rodney back.

The DUI thing was hanging over my head, though. My dad told me I should plead not guilty and fight the charges in court. But I didn't have the guts. The judge sentenced me to DUI school, made me go to three Alcoholics Anonymous meetings, and had me pay a fine of $800—which to me, at that time, living on government checks, was a huge amount of money.

In other words, the judge convinced me that I couldn't really afford to continue drinking.

Barbara took this *very* seriously. She laid down the law. She said, "We have to get cleaned up. We can't stay together unless you quit drinking and I quit using drugs."

Barbara had been into cocaine. She smoked marijuana. She knew it wasn't good for her, just like the drinking wasn't good for me. She saw it was time for us both to get clean.

And so we did. It wasn't that hard. We didn't go to rehab. We didn't go to detox. We just quit.

My life looked different to me when I wasn't drinking all the time. It didn't look good. It looked like it was going nowhere. I was an adult. I was a father. But I was sort of nothing, after that. I had never had a real job. I had never had anything like a career.

It's like I had been living in some kind of fog, and the fog started to lift. One day I woke up and realized I wasn't going anyplace. I was almost forty years old. I was ten years behind everyone I knew. I was just starting to do, in my late thirties, what most people had finished doing at twenty. I had been doing at twenty what most people did at ten. I felt out of place, and like my life was out of control.

I didn't like the way I was living. Christine was having a hard time making ends meet, and Justin and Rodney missed each other.

Barbara and I decided that the best way to take care of everybody was for us all to live together—again.

We rented a house on Curtner Avenue, in the Cambrian Park area of San Jose. It was a four-bedroom stucco place with a huge avocado tree in the side yard and a big old apple tree in the backyard. The front yard was filled with rose bushes, and the apple tree was full of rats. We had to cut the apple tree down to get rid of the rats.

We lived sort of hand-to-mouth. I had my government money. Christine was working. She had a job in the kitchen at Herman Sanitarium, a convalescent hospital for the mentally ill in San Jose. Barbara was still working at Our Lady of Fatima Villa.

I wasn't doing much of anything. But now, for the first time in my life, I was ashamed of that.

What was wrong with me? I was willing to accept that I was different, that something bad had been done to me. But I was sick of being a wannabe and a wannahave. All my adult life I had been living off the government and off women like Barbara and Chris. I felt like I owed it to my kids, and to the women I was living with, to do better.

So I enrolled at Phillip's College, a private school with a campus right near where we were living, and started taking classes in computer science.

It was a little scary. This was 1991. I was forty-three years old, and I was surrounded by kids twenty years younger than me. I hadn't been in school since Rancho Linda—almost thirty years before. I was afraid I wouldn't make the mark.

Mostly, I did fine. In some classes, I did better than fine. I still have a couple of papers I wrote for my English 1A teacher, Mrs. Davis. One of them is called "A Blade of Grass."

"Somewhere there is a blade of grass that has been unchanged by man or machine," I wrote. "It will sprout forth, grow, and die, without ever being validated by man nor beast. How many butterflies in all their splendid glory are born and fly through a mountain meadow, and soon die without their beauty ever being viewed or appreciated?"

The teacher gave me an A and wrote on it, "This is lovely, Howard. It reminds me of Gray's 'Elegy.' "

I spent two years at Phillip's. In 1993 I graduated with an AS degree. I went out to look for a job as a computer repairman. I got some work doing that, but not a real job. It was mostly friends asking me if I could fix their Macs and PCs. They'd give me twenty dollars to replace the hard drive. It was a bad way to make a living.

I probably would have gone on like that, except that two things happened that turned my life upside down.

In early 1994, my grandma Boo died. She was ninety-six years old. She had been living alone in a house in Cupertino. One Sunday morning she made herself some breakfast, sat down in her favorite chair, turned on the TV, and died.

Five months later, I almost joined her. On July 7, 1994, I had a heart attack.

I woke up that morning with a stomachache. This was not that unusual. I lived a very unhealthy lifestyle. I smoked three packs of cigarettes a day. I drank coffee. I had bad eating habits. I would sometimes eat four or five Jack in the Box cheeseburgers as an afternoon snack, and then come home and eat a big dinner. I remembered having stomach pain the night before. I didn't think it was anything important.

But it got worse. Soon I was sweating, and I had the chills. I was getting hot flashes and cold flashes, and the pain was intense. Barbara said I should go down to this health clinic to get checked out.

I had already decided I wasn't having a heart attack. I was in denial almost as soon as I was in pain. I was sure this was nothing but stomach trouble.

The people at the clinic weren't so sure. They thought I should get a chest X-ray and an EKG. They wanted me to go to the hospital for the tests.

Well, I didn't feel *that* bad. I figured if I was having a heart attack, I'd know it. I remember leaving the clinic and having a cigarette. I thought, *If I can still smoke, it's not a heart attack, right?*

An hour later, I felt even worse. So we went to the hospital. The technicians gave me an EKG, then took me down to radiology. They hadn't even shot the first frame before these guys came running in and threw me into a wheelchair.

"It's serious," they said. "You're having a heart attack."

But instead of taking me into the ICU, they took me to the business office, where they made me and Barbara fill out a million forms.

I was really scared, and I was angry. I was going to die, and they were making me fill out a bunch of forms!

The doctors had me in the ICU for five or six days. The cardiologist told me a piece of fat had blocked one of the main arteries in my heart, but then had been pushed through and was no longer a problem. I should have died, but I was going to be all right.

My dad came to visit me. So did my boys. Chris came. They all rallied around.

I never smoked another cigarette. That one outside the clinic was the last one I ever had. The date of my heart attack is the day I quit smoking forever.

My recovery was slow. I didn't rush things. I had medical insurance. I had my monthly check. I was afraid of having another heart attack, and I used that as an excuse to not do anything.

But I made an important decision. If I was going to die from another heart attack, I wanted to be married to Barbara before I did.

The date was September 30, 1995. It was a big outdoor wedding. My dad came, and my new stepmother—Lois, who I liked a lot. My little brother Kirk was there, all the way from Washington, and my uncle Kenny, and his wife and family. I was sorry my grandma Boo wasn't still alive to see it. I'd have liked her to be there. My brother Brian didn't come. My stepbrother George didn't come, either.

Barbara's matron of honor was a friend from work. My best man was Edgar Rivera, a friend from college. All of Barbara's sisters came. So did her brother John—on his chopper, along with another guy from the Los Gatos chapter of the Black Watch motorcycle club. There were about forty guests in all.

Barbara wore a traditional white lace dress with long sleeves. I wore a tuxedo.

Barbara's employers at the convalescent hospital sent us on our honeymoon. They bought us four days and nights at the Monterey Plaza Hotel in downtown Monterey, in a big room right by the water. We ate breakfast in bed, overlooking the bay. We went for walks around the harbor. We rented one of those bicycle carts that can seat two or four or six. The bicycle-rental guys hung a sign on the back of the cart that said JUST MARRIED.

We came back to San Jose. I was out of work. I was still recuperating. But I couldn't take living with Chris anymore.

She had always brought home strays—*I* was one of them—and that was part of her charm. Her door was always open. But now her door was open to all kinds of people who we didn't want to live with us and the boys. The house was already a little crowded with five of us sharing it. Then Chris invited her sister Cindy to move in. Her husband, Henry, had committed suicide some years before, but Cindy still had two sons. So that made eight of us. Plus, all of the boys were welcome to have their friends around all the time. I'd get up in the morning and there'd be people I never saw before sleeping on the living room floor.

So Barbara and I rented a house in Saratoga, near where Barbara had grown up. Chris stayed in the house on Curtner with Justin and Rodney.

Chris had changed jobs again, too. She was back at Our Lady of Fatima Villa, working with Barbara. She had never been the picture of good health, but one day at work she had an episode. She had pain in her left side, and she couldn't lift her left arm.

She insisted it was just a muscle pull, and she refused to see a doctor.

But then she had a second episode, and it was more serious. She almost died. She wound up in the hospital on a ventilator. They did all the tests and discovered that she had a very advanced case of hardening of the arteries. She had 90 percent blockage in her heart, and only one valve was working properly. She was too unhealthy and weak for them to operate. She was a heavy smoker—two packs a day for years—and she was overweight, and she had a history of heart disease in her family. The doctors told her she had six months to live.

Rodney and Justin were both in high school. They weren't doing too good either. They had discovered crystal methamphetamine, and they liked it, and they were both really into it. They had a dealer who lived right down the street. They'd just trot over there when they ran out and get some more.

Maybe the boys didn't realize how sick their mother was. Maybe it was the drugs. They didn't really understand that they were living with a woman who might die at any time. But she was getting weaker and weaker. She had stopped showering because she had this terrible fear of dying in the shower. Her leg was turning black from lack of circulation, and she knew what that meant. She had worked in convalescent hospitals for a long time. She knew a lot about sickness and death.

But she didn't seem scared. She had always had this dream when someone close to her was about to die. It was a dream about bread and fish—something about being at work in the hospital kitchen, and running out of bread and not having enough food to feed everyone. She had that dream several times when people she worked with had died. Two of the hospital cooks had died of cancer, and one had had a heart attack, and she had the dream all three times right before they died.

Now she had the dream again, and she knew it was her turn.

One day she was worse than usual. The boys were at home.

Rodney could see she was in bad shape. He leaned down and held her for a while, but he didn't realize she was dying until she was dead.

He and Justin called 911 and the paramedics came right away. They were able to revive her twice. But she couldn't hold on. She died on the way to the hospital. She was fifty.

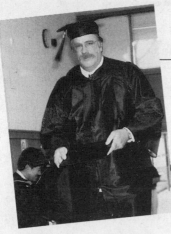

Chapter 14

Journey

With Chris gone, I had to get serious about taking care of my children. It was time for me to grow up and start living like a regular citizen. But I couldn't get work in the area I was trained for. I remember thinking, *Why did I bother getting this degree when they won't even give me a job? I might as well drive a bus.*

So that's what I did. I got a job driving a bus.

For the first time in my life, it was a real job. Christine's sister Cindy was working for a company that supplied bus drivers for IBM. She got me in. Soon I was driving a Blue Line bus around the huge IBM plant, taking workers here and there. I liked the work. I had to wear black pants and a white shirt, which I didn't like so much, but I also got to wear an IBM identification badge. That was pretty snooty.

It was a long workday every day. I went to work at six in the morning and got off at six at night—if I was lucky. Sometimes I had to work nights, or weekends. The law says you're not supposed to do that. You're not allowed to do any kind of driving, for safety reasons, for more than ten hours a day. That's what those log books that truckers keep are all about, to prove they haven't driven more than ten hours a day. The authorities don't want to have sleepy drivers behind the wheel, especially if they're driving other people around.

Besides that, I liked the driving. I liked the people. I liked learning to get along with them. This was a new thing for me. In jail, and at Agnews, and at Rancho Linda, even though I was surrounded by people, I didn't have to get along with them. My size always took care of that for me. Now I had to learn how to deal with people as equals.

I stayed at IBM for a couple of years. I was making okay money. But I started getting pretty burned out. I was living a pretty unhealthy lifestyle. I didn't drink or smoke anymore, but I never exercised, and I wasn't careful about what I ate. The hours were killing me. Sometimes on Friday night, when I was exhausted and ready to take the weekend off, I'd be told I was scheduled to make some more runs on the weekend.

When I couldn't take it anymore, I quit and applied for a job with a tour-bus company called Serendipity. I thought it would be better if I was driving a tour bus. The pay was okay, and they seemed to need drivers. I went in and applied on a Friday, and they told me to report for work the next Monday. Then, when I had barely gotten home from the job interview, they called and said I had to come back right away—they already had a run for me.

That should have told me something. They didn't have enough drivers. The Serendipity job turned out to be as rough on me as the IBM job. The hours were too long. The stress was too much for me.

So I quit.

A little later I started up again at another company, this time an outfit called Durham, which mostly supplied buses for schools. It was a good company. It had a good vibe. The company wasn't choking on a lot of regulations. But they took the bus driving seriously, and all the drivers were properly licensed, and all the mechanics were ASC-certified.

Durham ran about eighty or ninety buses every day. They supplied buses for the special-education kids at the San Jose schools and the West Valley schools, and all the buses for the Cambrian Park schools, where my boys went when they were little. They had other buses going out to Monterey and Santa Cruz. It was a busy company.

Sometimes I drove regular kids, and sometimes I drove special-education kids. I liked the special-ed kids better. The regular kids acted like special-ed kids—or the way you'd *think* special-ed kids would act, all immature and out of control. They were little maniacs. Fortunately, I was only with them for ten or fifteen minutes at a time. Besides, if you're six feet seven inches and as big as I am, all you have to do is stand up and the kids get quiet.

But I did yell at a kid one time, and got his mom mad at me. He was a fifth-grader, and I asked him why he was behaving worse than the kindergarten kids. His mom came in the next day and told me I had embarrassed her son in front of his friends. I told her I thought he *should* be embarrassed, but I apologized—sort of. I said, "Next time he's upset, instead of yelling at him in front of his friends, I'll make an appointment to discuss the problem with him over coffee and doughnuts." She didn't like that much.

I don't think I identified with the special-ed kids, but I felt for them. I used to look at them and get sad. I'd realize that this little girl was never going to get married or have kids, or that boy was never going to be able to run or jump or play basketball.

Sometimes I would look at a kid and think, *There, but for the grace of God, go I.* If those needles had gone a little deeper, or if they'd twirled a little differently one direction or the other, it might have been *me* riding the short bus.

Anyway, I liked being around them. I grew attached to them. Remember, with some of these kids, you drive them five days a week, every week, for a whole school year—and then maybe the next year, too. You get to know them, and you get to like them. That wasn't so true with the regular school kids. I didn't *want* to know most of them.

My life leveled out. I was working. My health was better. My head was clearer. I began to see my life differently. I began to think about my life, and about what had happened to me, in a new way—not so emotional, more analytical.

This made me helpful to others, just as it made me helpful to myself. When Barbara's sister Linda was arrested and jailed for drugs, I decided to go visit her. I knew a little about drugs, and I knew a lot about jail. I thought I could help. She was locked up at the Santa Cruz county jail. I arranged to go visit her.

I knew what it was to be locked up. I knew what you thought about, and what you missed, and what you were afraid of when you were inside. So I was able to talk to her. I told her she had to make a decision. She had to quit drugs. She had to stop throwing her life away. I told her it was up to *her* to have a decent life. No one was going to give it to her. She had to do it herself.

I visited her every Sunday, without Barbara ever knowing, for about two months. Something I said must have sunk in. She got out of jail, and went to live with some friends. She quit using drugs. She went to Bethany College in Scotts Valley, and got a degree. She became a drug counselor. She's still doing that work today.

As time passed and my life cleared up, I found myself thinking more and more about my childhood. There was a lot I didn't remember. There was a lot I didn't understand. In reality, I didn't really know what had happened to me, or why it had happened to me. I began to ask myself whether I had really been given a lobotomy. I wondered why I wasn't a vegetable, if what I knew about lobotomies was true. I began to wonder whether I had deserved one, and whose decision it had been to give me one.

These were questions I had never asked anybody—not my dad, not Lou, not Freeman, not the doctors at Agnews or the counselors at Rancho Linda. But now I started to ask.

The trouble was, most of the people who knew the answers were gone.

Grandma Boo had died. Freeman had died. Then Lou died, too, at the beginning of 2000.

She and my dad had divorced sometime before. He told me that she didn't like his dog, and that was the last straw. She was mean to his dog. I couldn't help thinking at the time, *She gives your son a*

*lobotomy, and that's okay. Then she's mean to your dog and you get a
divorce?*

My dad had married again, to Lois.

Lou had met a man named George Kitasako. He was born in
America to parents who had emigrated from Japan and then were
placed in internment camps in Wyoming during World War II. I
don't know how he and Lou met, but they were together for ten
years. My brother George said they were very happy.

George Kitasako died in 1988. Lou was on her own for the rest
of her life. She never lost her anger at my father for the way things
had turned out. My brother George thought she was poisoning
his children's minds against their grandfather, and he didn't like it.
She complained about him so often that he had to ask her to stop.

Lou spent her last days in a hospital in Portland, Oregon, where
she had moved to be near her oldest son, Cleon, after her friend
George died. Cleon came to sit with her every day for three months.
The nurses told him that she was a very strong woman, and that
she probably would not die while he was there. She would die in
her own way, when she was alone, when no one was watching.

That's what happened. Cleon had been there for part of New
Year's Eve. He was coming back on New Year's Day. They called
him before he arrived, early on January 1, and told him she had
died in the night.

There was an obituary in the Mountain View paper. It said,
"Lucille Jackson, a longtime resident of Los Altos and Mountain
View, died January 1. A native of San Francisco, she was 80. Mrs.
Jackson was a graduate of Mountain View High School. She
trained as a medical assistant at Foothill College. She is survived by
children, Cleon M. Cox, George Cox, Howard Dully, Brian Dully
and Kirk Lee Dully and many grandchildren."

I told my dad I wanted to go to her funeral. Even though I had
hated her, and I had been afraid of her, she was an important part of
my life. She was "Mom" to me longer than my real mother was. I
thought it was right that I should go and pay my respects.

My father saw it differently. He told me I would upset people if I went. He said it would make people think about what had happened to me, and take the focus off Lou and the funeral and the mourning. So, I didn't go.

My dad's health was okay, but then he got sick, too. Or, he found out he was sick, kind of by accident.

His brother had a massive heart attack and nearly died. My dad went in to have his own heart checked, and found out he was in danger of a heart attack himself. So he had quadruple bypass surgery not long after that.

He recovered fine. But I realized that he wasn't going to be around forever. If I was going to find out more about what happened to me, I was going to have to start investigating. I needed to understand my past now. I needed it for my future.

So I started doing research on the Internet. I'd go to a search engine, and I'd type in the word *lobotomy*, and I'd start reading. I learned about the operation. I learned that Freeman was the most famous guy who ever did it. I found out why it wasn't used anymore. I read some case histories on people who'd had lobotomies. But I couldn't find out anything about lobotomies on children, and I couldn't find out anything about *me*.

Then, one day about a year after I started doing the research, I came upon a reference to a book called *Great and Desperate Cures* by Elliot S. Valenstein, about all the ways that doctors had tried to cure or treat mental illnesses. There was a lot about lobotomy, and about Freeman.

And on page 274, there was something about me.

Valenstein told a story about Freeman going to the Langley Porter Clinic in San Francisco to make a presentation about lobotomy in young adults, and bringing with him three young people—including a twelve-year-old boy—who had been given transorbital lobotomies. It was January 1961. That twelve-year-old boy was me.

I don't know why it mattered to me that I found this book. I'd already known I had been to Langley Porter. I'd known Freeman was my doctor. I'd been pretty sure he'd given me a lobotomy. But seeing it in print made it real.

I kept researching. I started doing searches for *lobotomy and children*. I figured someone, somewhere—with all the universities and hospitals and newspapers and magazines out there—*had* to be interested in lobotomy in children. Somebody was probably studying it, and would want to talk to a guy like me.

I wrote to hospitals that specialized in brain surgeries. I contacted psychiatric hospitals and institutions. Nobody answered. Nobody was interested. Or, if they were, I couldn't find them. But I did find a Web site called psychosurgery.org, run by a woman named Christine Johnson. She had created the Web site to start a discussion about lobotomy and other methods doctors were using to change people's personalities by operating on their brains. The Web site had a blog that contained all kinds of information about lobotomy—history, news, events, lawsuits, whatever. (You can go on and learn, like I just did, that at a recent meeting of the Institute of Psychiatry at King's College in London, transorbital lobotomy was officially awarded the title of worst psychiatric treatment ever conceived. Thank you, King's College.)

Christine introduced me, by e-mail, to a woman named Carol Noell. Her mother had been lobotomized. She and Christine were both doing research on the procedure, and on Freeman. They offered to introduce me to people who were interested in lobotomy. One of them, the same Dr. Valenstein who had written about Freeman's work, finally responded to me. He said I should drop my research and get on with my life. What happened was a long time ago. If you're okay now, and you're happy, he said, you should just forget about it.

That wasn't a satisfactory answer. So I kept going.

A little later, Christine told me she had heard about a radio producer who was preparing some kind of radio report on Walter Freeman. She asked if she could give him my name and phone number.

I was a little hesitant. I wanted information, but I didn't want to *give* information. I didn't want to be part of any radio show. But I told Christine she could give the producer my e-mail address.

Sometime in the fall of 2003 I was contacted by a person named Piya Kochhar. We chatted. She was nice. She was from India. She told me she was working on this project about Walter Freeman.

She told me her partner was an important radio producer named Dave Isay. Dave had become fascinated with lobotomies after visiting Greystone, the famous old insane asylum in upstate New York. Then he read a story about Freeman in the *Wall Street Journal*, written by a man named Jack El-Hai, who was working on a biography of Freeman. Using Jack's help, Dave and Piya started trying to contact some of Freeman's former patients. That led him and Piya to Christine, who led them to me.

I told Piya about my lobotomy. But I also told her I was concerned about participating in a radio show, because of the stigma attached to lobotomy. Piya reassured me. She said, "We're doing a radio documentary on Walter Freeman, not on you." But she did want to interview me. She and Dave wanted to come to California to speak with me in person.

I was flattered. I would have been more flattered if I had known more about her partner, and what kind of work he did.

I don't listen to National Public Radio all that much. I'm more of a golden-oldies FM-radio type guy. I hadn't heard of Sound Portraits, which was Dave's radio production company. So I didn't know he had been awarded a Guggenheim Fellowship and a MacArthur Fellowship, and had won four Peabody Awards—which is like winning four Pulitzer Prizes, or four Oscars, for radio—plus a bunch of other awards. Even though he was still a young guy, he was already a kind of legend in radio. He was also the founder of StoryCorps, which is a team of radio producers that tours the country getting ordinary people to tell the dramatic stories of their lives. Since 2003 they've helped hundreds of everyday Americans interview their parents, or grandparents, or great-grandparents, and document their personal histories.

I didn't know anything about this. All I knew was that there was someone out there who was very, very interested in hearing me talk about my lobotomy. At last, there was someone who cared enough about what happened to me to ask me some intelligent questions. And I was really impressed that they were going to get on a plane and come all the way from New York just to talk to me.

In the fall of 2003 I was still working for Durham. In 2000, I had started training bus drivers. In 2003, I became state certified as a behind-the-wheel instructor. I was making better money than I'd ever made before, and I liked the work.

Barbara and I were living in Aptos at the time, in an apartment near the beach that had a nice view of Monterey Bay. In preparation for Dave and Piya's visit, Barbara and I got the place all cleaned up. We took all the junk from the living room and the dining room and stashed it in the bedroom. We didn't want them to think we were untidy people. We sat in the window staring out, waiting for them to come. I was so nervous that I had to go sit outside on the landing and wait for them.

When they pulled into the parking lot and started walking up, I remember being a little shocked. Here was this big tall guy, carrying a notepad or something, and behind him was this small woman, carrying a huge amount of radio gear. To a man of my generation, that's just not right. You don't make the *girl* carry everything. I didn't realize Piya was working for Dave, that she was in charge of all the radio equipment, and this was her job.

They had brought gifts. Somewhere in our discussion I must have told Piya that Barbara collected snow globes, because she had brought one for her. We invited them in and we all sat around the living room, talking, getting to know each other.

In person, just like on the phone, Piya was comfortable to be with. Dave was not as easy. He was very nice, but he had this habit of always moving his eyes around, always looking around the room, like he was searching for something. It made me a little uneasy.

Then, when it was time to do the interview, Dave said he wanted to see our bedroom. That's where all the junk was. I didn't want him to go in there. But he said the interview had to be done there, because that was always the quietest room in the house. So we went in. Dave sat in a chair at the side of the bed. Barbara and I sat on the bed. Piya sat at the foot of the bed, holding a big boom microphone.

I don't remember what Dave asked me. I know I talked about my operation, and my family, and how things went wrong in my family. I was nervous. Dave had a notebook on his lap, and he would make notes with a pencil, and sometimes he'd interrupt me and ask a question. "How did that make you feel?" or "What happened after that?"

After a while we took a break. We decided to get some dinner. We went to a good Mexican place right near our house. After dinner, Dave and Piya went back to their hotel.

Sometime in the night after that dinner, they made a decision. They loved my story. They loved my voice. They decided to drop Walter Freeman as the subject of their documentary. They were going to make their documentary about *me*.

The next day, they played to my vanity. They told me I had such a beautiful voice and such good radio "presence" that they wanted to tell the story of Walter Freeman by telling the story of *my* lobotomy. They wanted me to interview all the doctors, nurses, and patients they could find. I would be the voice on the radio interviewing all these people.

I agreed. But I had a few rules. I would not let them use my last name. I would not get on an airplane. I would not interview my father.

They agreed to my conditions. We began. And almost immediately I had to change my mind about the rules I had set down.

First, they wanted me to come to Atlanta, to interview a woman and her mother. The mother had been a lobotomy patient, and the woman had agreed to let her be interviewed. But I didn't want to fly.

They also wanted me to interview my father. Piya kept harping on this, but in a nice way. She'd say, "We really think we should interview your dad," or, "We really think it would be good if you interviewed your dad." I just kept saying, "I don't want to do that." I never refused, exactly, and she never insisted. I just kept saying that I didn't want to do it, and she kept coming back to it.

My problem was that I didn't want my dad to get upset with me. Our relationship was not great, but at least I had him in my life again. I was afraid that if I told him about the documentary he'd get mad and disown me, or threaten to never speak to me again.

In early 2004, Dave and Piya called with some important news. They had contacted George Washington University in Washington, D.C., where Freeman had donated all his professional papers, and discovered that the archives were open to anyone who had been one of Freeman's patients. I could ask to see everything Freeman had on me—notes, documents, photographs, everything. But I had to come to Washington in person. The records couldn't be released any other way. I had to come right away, and I had to fly.

I really didn't want to. Not because I don't like flying. It's because I'm *afraid* to fly. Really afraid.

I've always felt that way. So, because I'm not stupid enough to do things that scare me, I had never been on a plane. But I've seen the airplane crashes on TV. I figured, if I'm not on the plane, I don't have to worry about it crashing.

The other problem is I'm a little claustrophobic. I don't like to be in confined spaces. And a guy my size on an airplane is automatically in a confined space. I wouldn't be able to curl up and go to sleep, like some people do when they fly. So that means I would be wide awake, and scared, every minute of the flight.

I know it's not completely logical. But that doesn't change the way I feel. When I'm on the ground, in a car or on a bus or a train, I feel like I'm in control. I can get out. Plus, I understand how they work. I don't understand the plane. I just can't understand the logic of this giant building up in the air, flying around with people in it. It doesn't make sense.

But Dave and Piya were insisting. They needed me in Washington, D.C., to get to the archives. They needed me in Atlanta, Georgia, to do that interview. There wasn't time for me to take the train.

There was also the question of the expense. Dave's production company had frequent flier miles with Delta Airlines, so I could fly to the East Coast and back for free. If I was going to take the train, and get a sleeper, and get my meals taken care of, it would take three days and a lot of money to do what we could do in a few hours, and for free, on an airplane.

I didn't care about any of that. But I cared about the archives. I wanted to see what was in there. I wanted to see it so badly that I even agreed to get on an airplane.

I tried to psych myself into thinking it was all going to be okay. Why wouldn't it be okay? People fly all the time. It was going to be fine.

It wasn't fine. Barbara and I went to the airport. We had planned to take the red-eye to Atlanta, so I wouldn't have to look out the window and see how high up we were. I took some melatonin to help me sleep, and some Xanax. Neither one of them worked. I was wide awake and scared to death the whole trip.

We landed about five in the morning. I understood why they called it the red-eye.

But I didn't have too much time to feel sorry for myself. Dave and Piya met us at the hotel lobby early the next morning. We had some breakfast and went to work.

Our first interview was with Ann Krubsack, a woman who had been lobotomized by Freeman at Doctors General Hospital a week after me.

To my surprise, and disappointment, her feelings about Freeman, and her lobotomy, were all completely positive. This little, round, silver-haired woman thought he was a great man and the operation was a wonderful thing.

We got something different during the second interview, with Carol Noell.

She's the woman I had met on the Internet a couple of years before, through the Web site psychosurgery.org. In person, she was an attractive, light-haired woman. She suffered from MS, so she moved a little slowly.

She had suffered from a lot more than that as a child. Her mother, Anna Ruth, was lobotomized by Freeman in 1950, after being treated for a series of crippling headaches. The procedure cured Carol's mother of her headaches. It also left her with the mind of a child. And, like a child, she was carefree and without anxiety of any kind. Carol never had a real mother after that.

Piya set up the microphones and recording equipment. I started asking the questions I had worked out with Dave. Carol was easy to interview. She had a story to tell about her mother, and she was ready to tell it.

"Did she worry about stuff?" Carol said. "Nope. Didn't worry. Just as Freeman promised . . ."

But she also had "no social graces," Carol said. If she was out walking and saw people getting together for a party, or sitting down to dinner, she'd walk right into their home and make herself comfortable—even if they were people she didn't even know.

"She was the greatest playmate we ever had, and the best friend, and we all loved her to death," Carol said. "But I never called her Mama, or Mommy, or anything. I never even thought of her as my mother, or as my daughter's grandmother. And I never even took my daughter to see her. . . ."

It was a heartbreaking story, and a very emotional interview for me. This was the first time I had met someone whose life had been damaged, like mine, by a lobotomy. It wasn't Carol's surgery, but it affected every day of her life after it took place.

We left Carol Noell and drove the rest of the day to Birmingham, Alabama. By the time we got there, we were all exhausted. We got rooms in a Holiday Inn, and after dinner finally got some rest.

The next morning we met with Rebecca Welch. Her mother, Anita McGee, had been suffering from severe postpartum depression when she was lobotomized by Freeman in 1953. The lobotomy had relieved her depression, but left her distant and disconnected.

"She's there, but she's not there," Rebecca said to me.

Rebecca's mother had lived in a nursing home for many years, and Rebecca had dutifully visited her, every single week. But she never told anyone about her mother. She never talked about the lobotomy, like it was some kind of shameful secret. In fact, in the nineteen years she had been married, Rebecca had never once taken her husband to meet her mother.

We were scheduled to meet Rebecca at the nursing home. When we arrived, we were taken into a little side room where Rebecca and her husband were waiting. Rebecca was a slender blonde with long curly hair and a strong southern accent. We said our hellos, and spent a few minutes getting to know each other, while Dave and Piya prepared their recording equipment.

Then they wheeled Rebecca's mother in on a sort of gurney.

She was in bad shape. She tried to talk, but she couldn't. When she spoke, it sounded like she was gargling. I couldn't understand anything she said. We tried to talk a little but it was no good.

So Rebecca had her sing something instead. She said, "What was that song, Mom? Remember?"

Together, they began singing "You Are My Sunshine."

After her mother had been taken away, Rebecca said, "I don't know who could have perceived this procedure as a miracle cure. The only thing I see that came out of it was hurt and pain for a lot of people."

I asked her why she had waited so many years to bring her husband to meet her mother.

"It's been so painful that I've tried to stay very far away from it for a long time," she said. "Kind of like, if you leave it alone, it will go away. But it never goes away."

"What has changed your mind about hiding from it?"

"You," she said, and started to cry.

We both broke down. Through her tears, Rebecca told me I was helping people just by standing up and asking the questions I was asking.

"Do you know how many people you're championing?"

I hadn't thought of it that way. But hearing her say it helped me believe I was doing something worthwhile. I had been a little leery at times. Was I doing this the right way, going so public with it? Was I doing it for the right reasons? Was I being unfair, or vindictive?

Rebecca said, "You're like all those people who were locked away, who could not go on this quest, who could not ask all these questions. You're doing it for all of them."

That was very moving to me. We sat together and cried for long enough that Barbara started to feel a little left out. Rebecca and I had made a sort of bond. Like me, and like Carol, she had lost her childhood—not to her own lobotomy, but to her mother's. And like us she had this sense of pain and loss and outrage. And now she finally had met someone who understood that.

I felt stronger about the whole project after that interview. I felt like I could go through anything to get it finished if I was doing it in a way that was going to help other people. It would also heal me in ways I never could have seen ahead of time.

I felt strong enough to get back on an airplane, even. We drove the whole way back to Atlanta from Birmingham that afternoon, with barely enough time to ditch the rental car and get to the airport. We flew up to Washington, D.C., that night.

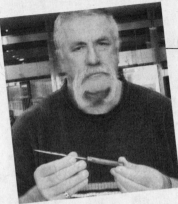

Chapter 15

Archives

We were up and out early the next morning. It was February. It was *cold*. There was snow on the ground. Barbara and I left our hotel escorted by Dave and Piya and their radio equipment, and headed for the archives.

The walk took us past the White House, down Pennsylvania Avenue, toward Washington Circle, until we got to George Washington University. It's a stately campus, full of trees and historic red-brick buildings. The archives room was in a big, square, modern building with a lot of glass.

The university archivists, led by a guy named David Anderson, took us up to the second floor to a brightly lit room with glass walls and sleek furniture. They were ready for us. There, on a table, was a folder with my name on it. Out of the twenty-four individual boxes of private papers, notes, correspondence, photographs, and published work that Freeman had donated to the university, this was the folder on *me*.

Piya and Dave asked me to sit at the table in front of the folder, but told me not to open it until they were ready. They set up their recording equipment. Then Dave took the folder and began studying the documents. He wanted to see them before I did, he said, so he could have an idea of what was coming. He wanted to be ready to record my reactions and ask me follow-up questions.

I was nervous—nervous and kind of scared. In that folder was the evidence. This was the proof. The papers inside held the answers to the questions that had been plaguing me for more than forty years: Why did they do this to me? What did I do to deserve it? Was I going to find out I had been an ax murderer or something?

I was the first Freeman patient, and maybe the first lobotomy patient, ever to come forward to see his case history. But the archivists were prepared. There were several boxes of tissues on the table beside the folder. The archivists were ready for someone to do some crying.

Piya held the boom microphone. Dave turned on the recording equipment. One by one, he began handing me things from the folder.

First came the pictures. There were three eight-by-ten black-and-white pictures of me on the operating table. There were before, during, and after pictures—of my face, my head with the needles sticking out, my face bruised and swollen.

They were pretty brutal.

In the before picture, shot with the camera looking straight at me, I'm wearing a hospital gown but the surgery hasn't started. I'm alert, and calm, and maybe a little defiant. There's something about the set of my jaw and the look in my eyes that says, "Okay, show me what you've got." I think it must have been taken the day I was admitted, the day before the operation.

In the during picture, I'm lying flat on my back. The photograph was taken of my profile, from my left side. My hair is brushed back off my forehead. My mouth is open. A man's left hand, with a hairy arm and a shiny wristwatch, is holding one end of a leucotome. The other end is sunk into my left eye socket. It looks like about three inches of the leucotome is actually in my skull.

In the after picture, the photograph was taken straight on again, perhaps by someone standing over me. I'm either asleep or passed out. I look like I'm dead. My face is swollen and my eyes are just slits in my face.

The pictures were not that upsetting to me. They were really graphic, and gruesome, but they didn't contain any new information. I pretty much knew what they did to me in that hospital. I knew what happened because of it. But I didn't know *why*. The pictures didn't tell me anything about *why*.

Dave and Piya and their researchers had already seen some of Freeman's archives. Those twenty-four boxes of his material contained similar photographs and similar documents on all the men and women Freeman had lobotomized over the decades. Freeman was an archivist's dream. He saved everything—case files on literally hundreds and hundreds of his patients. Most of the files had photos of the patients. There were before, during, and after pictures of them all.

According to Dave and Piya's research, the highest percentage of the patients were women. Some of the after pictures showed them recovering, on vacation, or posing with their husbands or boyfriends or families. The progression from first picture to last was not always an improvement. Some of the patients looked more disturbed in the after pictures than in the before ones. Others seem to span decades. Some of them begin as young women and finish as graying old crones.

Some of the photos were accompanied by holiday greeting cards, or newspaper clippings about the patient's activities. A lot of the patients appeared to be writing in response to something they'd received from Freeman. These letters began by saying, "Thank you for your recent card," or something like that.

Some patients were writing to report on their health. Others wanted marital advice. A surprising number talked about the weather. I thought that was weird. If you were exchanging letters with the doctor who had penetrated your brain with an ice pick, why would you write about having had a lot of rain this summer?

Other boxes contained holiday cards from former patients, each with a handwritten note indicating whether the patient had undergone a lobotomy or a transorbital lobotomy, and when. A woman named Onoria, of Harrodsbury, Kentucky, appears to have been

Freeman's ninetieth lobotomy patient. She wrote on a Christmas card, "How often we think of you—and how we were directed to you. God gave you a wonderful brain and skill. I feel good and am thankful I was saved. . . ."

Another woman, named Adelle, appears to have been Freeman's 537th lobotomy patient and then his 43rd transorbital patient. In 1958, she wrote to thank Freeman for his recent greeting card but went on to complain that "negros were crowding in to the neighborhood" where her sister was building a house. Three years later, a handwritten note explained that Adelle had moved in with the sister. Three years later still, the holiday greeting card was from the sister, not the patient. In the final note, the sister thanked Freeman for his message of condolence. Adelle had died.

Freeman followed some patients to the grave, and beyond. One file contained a newspaper obituary of a man identified as a "nylon stocking pioneer." A handwritten notation over his name reads "LOB 384." Freeman must have been proud of this patient. He clipped several of his obits.

In response to the cards and letters, Freeman was always upbeat and chatty. "I am retired now and enjoying hikes in the neighboring hills," he wrote to one former patient in 1967—the year he was finally forced to stop performing lobotomies. "If the end of the world does come soon, I shall have had my fun."

Dave and Piya hadn't brought me to Washington, D.C., to look at Freeman's files on other patients. They had brought me there to look at the files on *me*. So, when he thought I was ready, Dave began to hand me, one by one, papers out of the Howard Dully file, and asked me to begin reading them out loud.

The first one, dated October 5, 1960, began like this: "Mrs. Dully came in to talk about her step-son who is now 12 years old and in the 7th grade. The first time Mrs. Dully saw the boy she thought he was a spastic because of his awkward swing of his arms in walking and a peculiar gait. He doesn't react either to love or to punishment. He objects to going to bed but then sleeps well. He watches his chances and is clever at stealing. . . ."

I didn't really like seeing this in black and white, laid out in a doctor's reports, but it wasn't very surprising. I knew Lou thought these things about me. She had *yelled* these things at me for years. She was always accusing me of stealing things, of being clumsy, of being stupid. Well, I knew the truth about that. I wasn't stupid, and I wasn't clumsy. It was a little embarrassing to read out loud, but it wasn't anything new.

There was more. I was mean to my brother Brian. I didn't play well with the other boys. I teased the dog. I scowled at anyone who tried to change the channel when I was watching my favorite TV show, and most of my favorite TV shows featured violence. I did a lot of daydreaming. I was defiant. I didn't like to wash, and sometimes when I was younger I made a mess in my underpants.

That wasn't very surprising, either. I remembered being yelled at or punished for all these things. If Lou was going to complain about me to a doctor, that's what she would complain about.

Freeman didn't seem impressed. He didn't write anything about giving me a lobotomy, or considering me a candidate for a lobotomy. On October 18, 1960, two weeks after Lou's first visit, he wrote, "I declined to give any statement until I've seen Howard, and said I would have to see Mr. Dully first."

That caught my eye. Freeman declined to give any statement? Statement about what? And to whom? And he would have to see my dad first? First before what?

Were he and Lou already planning something?

Dave and Piya were recording me as I read each page. Barbara was watching me. The notes were harder for her than they were for me. She was crying already.

I wasn't crying at all. So far, this was exactly what I had expected—Lou telling lies to Dr. Freeman. There was nothing in the notes to indicate I was anything but a typical kid whose stepmother didn't like him.

But the notes and Lou's campaign against me continued. Freeman reported on November 30 that "things have gotten much worse and she can barely endure it." I was tormenting the dog, sticking pins in my little brother, and suffering from delusional ideas that everyone was against me. I was stealing things, maybe by breaking into houses along my paper route. Lou had to keep me separated from my brothers constantly, "to avoid something serious happening."

Freeman had a solution. Here, for the first time, he makes his diagnosis—"essentially a schizophrenic"—and suggests the treatment—"changing Howard's personality by means of transorbital lobotomy."

Well, there it was, in black and white. Freeman says, out loud, that I need a lobotomy.

I looked back at the top of the page. The date on that entry was November 30, 1960. It was my birthday. Lou was in Freeman's office, conspiring to turn me into a vegetable, making the decision that would rob me of my childhood and make a normal life impossible for me. And she was doing this on my twelfth birthday.

I got a little choked up. I got mad. I got emotional. It was hard for me to believe that anyone, even Lou, would treat a kid like this on his birthday.

But there it was. Lou didn't argue. She didn't ask to have the surgery explained. She agreed to go forward. Freeman said he'd meet with my dad.

Freeman did, the very next day. His notes for December 1 say he spoke to my dad and told him that I was a schizophrenic and that something had to be done right away. My dad agreed to go home and talk it over with Lou.

The next entry was dated two days later. "Mr. and Mrs. Dully have apparently decided to have Howard operated on; I suggested they come in for further discussions and not tell Howard anything about it."

Did my dad know what he was agreeing to? Did he know what a lobotomy was? Did Freeman explain what would happen to me? Did he tell my father that his firstborn son could wind up a vegetable, or *dead*? Did he say I might be a zombie? Or did he tell him—the way he seems to have told all his patients—not to worry because everything was going to be fine?

Sitting at the table in the archives room, I felt overcome by a terrible sense of abandonment and betrayal. Two days? It only took two days? My father thought about letting Freeman give me a lobotomy, and then gave his permission after only two days?

I felt overwhelmed. My hands were shaking. Barbara was crying. Piya was holding the boom mike. Dave was asking me occasional questions. The room was quiet. Below us, through the windows, I could see the snowy streets of Washington, D.C.

Dave continued to look through documents and hand them to me, one by one. I went back to reading.

Then I found the big lie.

It was just another page of Freeman's notes. But there was something wrong with it. The date was wrong. The first entry was dated November 30, 1960. The second and third were dated December 1 and December 3—the dates that my dad visited Freeman and then made his decision.

But the next entry was dated November 7, 1960. It was on the same page as the previous dates, but this date was out of order.

"Mr. Dully came in with Mrs. Dully today to talk over Howard's forthcoming operation," Freeman wrote.

> I learned from Mrs. Dully, when Mr. Dully was out, that Howard is suspected of having beaten his baby brother nearly to death since the infant was found in its crib with its skull fractured and its chest caved in and was barely saved from death. Mrs. Dully says she heard this from Mrs. Heaton who claimed that Mr. Dully himself had told her of it at the time of his wife's death; he said Howard hated the baby which he identified with the death of his mother; since Howard was only five years old at the time this seems rather likely.

What? Me? Beat my baby brother Bruce? It was a lie—a terrible, ugly lie.

Why was the entry dated wrong? Why had Lou told Freeman the story when my father was "out"? Why hadn't Freeman asked my father about it when he came back? He would have told him it wasn't true. Who was Mrs. Heaton? When had she told Lou this story? How could my father have told Mrs. Heaton the story "at the time of his wife's death," since she died when Bruce was only twelve days old?

And why—the biggest question of all—why had Lou waited so long to tell Freeman? For almost two months she had been trying to convince him that I was dangerous and crazy. If she believed I had beaten my infant brother nearly to death, why in the world would she have waited this long to tell it? Was she telling it now as a final nail in my coffin, to make sure Freeman had enough against me to justify a lobotomy?

Or had Freeman gone back and added this information *after* the lobotomy? Was he trying to protect himself by putting down some evidence to prove I was a lunatic? Was that why the date was wrong?

My head ached. I put the pages down. I got choked up. I couldn't go on reading.

For years and years I had wondered whether there was something I had done, some terrible crime I had committed, that made me deserve the lobotomy. There was a lot I had forgotten, a lot that was lost in the foggy aftermath of the surgery. Had I forgotten this, too? Was this the horrible thing I had done that made it necessary for them to hurt me?

Now I had the answer—and the answer was no. This was a lie. It was the biggest lie I ever heard. I never attacked Bruce. I *knew* that. He was a little infant, so retarded he didn't know his own name. Why would I hurt an innocent little baby like Bruce?

And why would Lou and Freeman conspire to hurt an innocent little boy like me?

I put the papers away and I broke down. I started crying. I said to Piya and Dave, "How is a twelve-year-old kid supposed to stand up to something like this?"

They turned off the recording equipment and gave me a few minutes to collect myself. I cried for a while.

It was terrible to read. That was *it*? That was all they had? That was all I had done? Even if it had all been true—and most of it, especially the things about me hurting Bruce, was lies—would it have justified my own family letting a doctor stick needles in my head and scramble up my brain?

When I had collected myself and we were done with the documents, the archivists asked if I wanted to see Freeman's tools. I said I did. Dave and Piya were surprised. They asked me several times if I was sure. Wouldn't it upset me to look at the doctor's instruments—to see, perhaps, the very leucotomes that had been used on me?

I said it wouldn't. They brought out the tools.

There was a whole box of them. Inside the box were about ten or fifteen instruments. One of them appeared to be the very first leucotome. It was the Uline Ice Company ice pick Freeman had used on his first patients. The others were more sophisticated variations, as Freeman did more and more lobotomies and perfected his technique. They were all made of heavy steel. They were about eight inches long. They had thick handles and sharp blades.

I held one in my hand. It was horrible to think a medical doctor would really stick this in a person's brain and slide it around.

But it didn't upset me to hold it. I felt its power, but I was not afraid of its power. I was no longer afraid of Freeman, or of what had happened to me. I had seen what they did to me, and why. It no longer had any power over me.

We left the archives building and walked back across the capital in the snow.

The following day, Dave and Piya took me to interview Dr. J. Lawrence Pool. He had been a colleague of Freeman's in the early part of his career.

There wasn't much I could ask him that related to me. He had known Freeman long before I came into the picture. Besides, he got angry at us during the interview. Dave kept asking him the same question, and asking him to say the same thing over and over again. In the broadcast, you could hear him say, "I dedicated my life to brain surgery," but it sounds like "braaaaiiiiin surgery," like he was Bela Lugosi, because Dave kept making him repeat the line.

But the interview was very helpful. Here was a medical colleague who was willing to say on the record that Freeman's methods offended him. "It gave me a sense of horror," he said. "How would you like to step into a psychiatrist's office and have him take out a sterilized ice pick and shove it into the brain over your eyeball? Would you like the idea? No!"

Dave and Piya seemed pleased. We had done good work. We had some good interviews in the bag. They were willing to let me and Barbara go back to California and recover.

Maybe now that there was no urgency, I could take my time heading home. My idea was to go slowly by train and see the country. I love to see things. Barbara and I have seen prairie dogs wave to us in Utah. I've seen elk standing by the tracks in Colorado. The time I spend on trains is a great opportunity to think, rest, do nothing, and work on my computer. I like to be alone just to think, and I don't get a lot of opportunity to do that. When I'm at work, I've got people around. When I'm home, after work, I've got family around. When I'm on a train, I have time to be alone and think.

But when it came time to go, we were given plane tickets and told when our plane was taking off. There wasn't time to argue about it.

It wasn't so bad. We met some people on the flight who were nice and understanding. They talked to me and calmed me down. It wasn't a bad flight. The plane didn't crash. I got home.

As soon as Barbara and I were back in California, Dave and Piya started talking to me again about interviewing my father. Because of what we had read in the archives, we *had* to interview him.

And it had to be me who did the interviewing. They were building the whole broadcast around me now, and everything depended on my voice. I had to interview my dad.

I didn't want to. I mean, I *really* didn't want to. I was afraid to.

But Dave and Piya were very persistent and very persuasive. I struggled with the decision for months, but I could see they were right. The radio program would be all wrong without it.

So that spring I wrote my dad a letter. Or, rather, Barbara wrote my dad a letter. I was trying, and I couldn't get anywhere with it. Barbara said she'd give it a shot and see what came out. What came out was beautiful:

Dear Dad,

I am writing you this letter because I know this is something that I know is hard to talk about for the both of us. I have gotten my records on the operation I had as a boy and I have some questions to ask. I have not asked them before this out of love for you, and I am afraid that asking will change your love for me. I was able to get the records by working with a company called Sound Portraits, and they are doing a story about me and others who have had this operation. I am the main character of the story.

I don't know if you know the complete story that was in the records, but I have interviewed people that have had the operation and doctors that could assess the operation. I would like to sit down with you and discuss what you know or feel about the operation. The records indicate that you were against it and that you basically were coerced into agreeing to have the operation done. The doctor that performed the operation was looking for someone of my age to perform the operation on and Lou was looking to fix something she felt was a problem. I know that I wasn't a perfect child, but the operation has haunted me all my life. Now that I am 56 years old, I need closure.

I have always loved you and would never do anything to hurt you. Please consider my need to discuss this and know that this is not about judging you as a father. This is just about under-

standing what happened to me as a child and how it has affected
me as a man.

Along with the letter, we sent copies of every single document from Freeman's archives. I photocopied everything. I wanted him to see the whole thing, and not think later that I had blindsided him.

I also sent him information on Dave Isay and Sound Portraits. I wanted him to know this wasn't some fly-by-night guy who was going to make "The Lobotomy Man from Mars." I wanted my dad to know this was a serious, award-winning radio documentarian.

Also, he needed to understand that we were going to make the documentary whether he participated or not.

I didn't have high hopes. Over the years I'd tried to ask my dad questions about what had happened to me. He was never willing to talk. His answers were always short and direct. He made it clear that the past was dead and buried and he wanted it to stay that way.

Four or five days later, we had an answer. My father sent me an e-mail. He said yes, he would be willing to talk with me. He said he didn't know how much he really remembered about that time, or what it was exactly we were going to ask him about, but he said yes.

This was a big surprise, and a big relief, but—this meant I was going to actually have to interview him. On some level, maybe I was hoping he'd say no and I wouldn't have to face him. Now I had to face him.

It was December 2004 before Dave and Piya could come back to California. They flew in, and we scheduled the meeting with my dad.

They had booked a room at the Pacific Hotel, on El Camino in Mountain View. Barbara and I met Dave and Piya there, and looked at the room where we were going to do the interview. Then Barb waited there while I went to pick up my dad.

It was only a few blocks, but it was a long ride. I hadn't seen my dad in several months, since before he had agreed to do the interview. Like I said, things between us hadn't been that tight. So the drive to the hotel was a little tense. I was on edge. I was nervous. My stomach was in knots. Did we talk? I can't remember. I told him I was glad to see him. I asked him about Lois and about his health. He seemed nervous, too. We didn't say anything about the subject at hand.

When we got to the hotel, we went straight into the interview. Dave and Piya recorded us greeting each other, like we hadn't said hello already. Then I made the introductions.

"I'm here with my dad," I said. "I've waited for over forty years for this moment. Thank you for being here with me."

"I'll tell you anything that needs to be answered," my dad said.

"Okay," I said. "We're here to talk about my transorbital lobotomy. How did you find Dr. Freeman?"

"I didn't. *She* did," he said. "She took you. I think she tried some other doctors who said, 'Nah, there's nothing wrong here. He's a normal boy.' It was the stepmother problem."

So, he was going to lay it all on Lou. I pressed him a little.

"My question would be, naturally, why would you let it happen to me, if that was the case?"

"I got manipulated, pure and simple," he said.

"Did you ever meet Dr. Freeman? What was he like?"

"I only met him, I think, the one time. He described how accurate it was, in that he had practiced the cutting on literally a carload of grapefruit. That's what he told me."

He laughed when he said that. I didn't tell him that Freeman had actually practiced on *cantaloupes,* which have more of the soft consistency of the human brain, and not grapefruit.

Dave had kept quiet so far, but I could see he was getting impatient. These weren't the answers he wanted. So he handed me a couple of photographs and told me to ask my dad to look at them.

"Have you ever seen a picture of the operation?" I asked him. "Would you mind if I showed you one?"

I gave him the picture of me on the table halfway through the operation, with the leucotome sticking out of my head.

He looked at it for the longest time. Then he said, "The thing

I'm intrigued by is how you look so *calm*. Maybe they gave you some medication."

"Electroshock treatments," I said.

"Oh!"

He kept looking at the picture. It seemed to have no effect on him at all. He said nothing.

Dave got even more impatient. He leaned forward and said, "How does it make you feel?"

"It's just a picture," he said.

Just a picture! It was his own son, but it made no impression. He started talking about where he was that day. He wandered off the topic.

Dave tried to bring him back. He said, "Can I ask you a couple of questions? Was Lou trying to convince you to do this? How did she convince you to do this?"

"I got manipulated," my dad answered. "I was sold a bill of goods. She sold me, and Freeman sold me, and I didn't like it."

Maybe so, but he sure didn't seem concerned about it now. None of this seemed to disturb him in any way.

So I asked him, "Is there anything in this that you regret at all?"

"See, that's negative," he said quickly. "And I don't dwell on negative ideas. And what am I talking about?"

"The positive."

"I always try to be positive."

I pushed a little further. On the tape, I sound like I'm begging him to listen to me, and to respond. "But this was, this has really affected my whole *life*."

"Nobody is perfect," he said. "Could I do it over again? Would I have? Oh, hindsight's beautiful. Fifty years later, can I say this was a mistake? So was World War One a mistake!"

Was that as far as he was willing to go—that a mistake was made? Forty years of my life had been lost, and the best he could do was agree that a mistake had been made? It hurt me to hear him say that. When I asked the question a different way, I started to get choked up.

"But I've had a lot of pain, during my life, because of the operation," I said. Then I started to cry. "I felt like a freak, a monster, a lot of the time, because of things I've seen and heard."

He seemed not to believe that. He wanted to know why people would make fun of me having a lobotomy, unless I told them I had a lobotomy. "How would they know?" he said.

I said that sometimes I'd just hear people making jokes—like the one about wanting to have "a bottle in front of me instead of a frontal lobotomy."

"Oh!" he said. "What you're saying is, it's like being a homosexual in a place that is totally nonhomosexual. And all you hear is antihomosexual jokes."

"Separated," I explained. "Different. For a long time I felt I was the only one. That I am the *only* one. This is what I've had to live with."

My dad got all positive on me again. "The one thing you have to do—it's up here that everything is," he said, pointing to his head. "And there isn't two of us alike on earth. We are *all* individuals."

I tried one more thing. I asked him, "Why do you think it's been so hard for us to talk about this?"

"You never asked about it," he said. "It was an unpleasant part of my life. I don't particularly want to delve into it. It's like, 'Let's go out and play in the horse manure.' But you were always able to talk to me. And you never did. I tried."

So his silence all these years was *my* fault. But he was willing to take a tiny bit of the blame.

"Maybe that's where I failed, in not letting you know I was able to be talked to," he said. "I was doing the same thing you were doing—waiting for me to put my hand out, as I was waiting for you to put your hand out."

His answers hurt me deeply, but I tried not to get defensive. I had asked him to come and he had come. I had asked him questions and he had answered. I didn't think I had any right to be angry with him for not giving me the answers I wanted.

"I want to thank you for doing this with me," I told him while the tape was still rolling. "I never thought this would ever happen."

"Well, you see? Miracles occur!" he said.

I had one more thing that I needed to say. I needed to say it out loud. I needed him to hear me say it.

"Actually," I stammered, "what I wanted to do was tell you that I love you."

This was a huge moment for me. I had never said that to my father, not once, my whole life. I was afraid to. I was afraid that if I said it to him he wouldn't say it to me.

Is this every kid's worst fear—that his mother and father don't love him? It was mine. Didn't my mother love me? She died and left me. Didn't my father love me? He let them cut my head open and hurt me. That's what I felt inside.

But I wasn't a kid anymore. I was old enough to understand that it didn't matter if he loved me, or said he loved me. It only mattered that I loved him, and that I said so.

I waited to hear him say he loved me, too. But he couldn't. He said, "Whatever made you think I didn't know that?" Then he added, "You shaped up pretty good!"

It wasn't "I love you, too," but it was enough. He was doing the best he could. I thanked him again for agreeing to talk with us on tape. We put the recording equipment away.

The following day, my dad and I met again, this time with a photographer Dave and Piya had hired to shoot some pictures of us. His name was Harvey Wang. He had been shooting pictures for all the interviews we did. Now he wanted to photograph me and my dad. He asked us if we could hug, so he could get a shot of that.

My dad refused. He said he didn't want to hug me. "I want to do that when I *want* to do that—not when it's some made-up thing for the camera."

So Harvey shot us standing next to each other, sort of smiling, sort of like old friends. You'd never know we were father and son, or that we'd been through any sort of ordeal.

We did many interviews over the next two months. We visited with Dr. Robert Lichtenstein, who had been Freeman's assistant on the day of my lobotomy. We also interviewed Freeman's sons—three of them, in three separate interviews.

Walter Freeman Jr. was the toughest. He's a neurobiologist at the University of California at Berkeley. He's a scientist. And he was very protective of his father. He was a difficult interview.

To tell you the truth, the interview creeped me out. He seemed like, from the way he was defending his father's work, he might have actually *continued* it, if he'd been given the opportunity. It worried me. This guy is part of the faculty at a medical school. He's responsible for shaping young minds. Does he tell them that lobotomy is a good thing?

Next we met Paul Freeman, in San Francisco. He invited us to his home. He had a friend with him, a French woman he identified as his roommate. He sat still for the interview, but I don't think we really learned anything new from him.

Then we met Frank Freeman, in San Carlos. He also welcomed us into his home. This was the first interview I did on my own, where I asked all the questions. I was nervous about it. I had a lot of anxiety. I guess it came down to this: Would people think I was a freak? Would they treat me like I was a freak? After all, when you hear that someone has had knitting needles stuck in their head and egg-beaten around for ten minutes, you might assume that they're going to be some drooling Frankenstein monster. I was afraid I might be treated that way.

Besides, I was in awe of Frank. As we were getting set up and ready to begin the interview, I could see his home was filled with books. When he spoke, I could hear he was very knowledgeable. He talked like a doctor, like he had complete knowledge of the operation and everything that went with it.

But he chuckled when he talked, in ways that were sort of creepy. He called the leucotome "the humble ice pick," and laughed. He

said that if he had a couple of leucotomes he could probably do a lobotomy right there in his house.

I was impressed by his apparent medical knowledge, but I was
upset by the interview. I got a bad headache. I found that I got a
bad headache after almost every single interview we did. I'm not a
guy who usually gets headaches. But when I'm under a lot of stress,
especially emotional stress, my head starts hurting me.

When we were finished, Dave asked Frank if he would mind
going into the other room and putting his work clothes on. I
thought this was weird. What work clothes? Why would Dave ask
him to do that?

He came back a few minutes later wearing his uniform. He was
a security guard! I thought he was a doctor, or a professor, or something connected to the medical field. But he worked as a security
guard. That blew me away. Frank and Dave got a good laugh over
it. I felt kind of foolish.

Dave and Piya went back to Brooklyn, to the Sound Portraits
studios, and began assembling the tapes. I went back to driving
school buses.

I didn't see my dad. I don't think I even talked to him. I was
worried that I had pushed him too far, that I'd made him uncomfortable, that he was mad at me for making him sit for the interview. But it was done. I couldn't take it back. The radio broadcast
was going forward.

I was still worried that he would ask me to stop it. I could imagine him telling me that it was a mistake, that I was going to hurt
the family, that I was being dishonorable to the memory of my
stepmother. I could imagine him telling me I had no right to do it.

That wouldn't have stopped the broadcast, but it would have
been difficult for me. I had never had a real confrontation with my
father after the lobotomy. There was never a single time after when
I stood up to him, or told him to leave me alone, or anything like
that. I never went up against him, face to face.

Maybe that's the problem. Maybe every boy needs to stand up to his dad one day and become his own man. But I never did that. So I was always afraid of him. Afraid of his anger. Afraid of his displeasure in me. I would like to call it respect—because that makes it sound honorable and manly—but it was really just fear. I wanted his approval. I spent most of my life trying to make him approve of me—and failing.

Did the operation do that? Did it make me less able to stand up for myself? Maybe there are people who, if the lobotomy had happened to them, would have been all over their fathers. "Why did you do this? How *could* you do this?" I could never ask those questions.

So I wasn't too happy to learn that Dave and Piya wanted me to interview my dad again. We didn't have enough. We didn't have him saying the things we needed him to say.

I let them contact him. I let them be the ones to ask for the second interview. Dave made the request. It was very casual. He said we just needed to clarify a few things, get a few details straight.

To my surprise, he agreed. But he had a stipulation. He said he hadn't been feeling too good. If he started to have pain during the interview, he'd have to stop.

The second interview took place the same way as the first one. Dave booked a room in the same hotel. I picked up my dad and drove him over.

Dave and Piya said hello, and got him comfortable in the room. Or tried to get him comfortable. He didn't seem well. He looked frail. His color wasn't good.

He's tall, like me—over six feet three inches—but he's thin. He's always been thin. Now he seemed even thinner and kind of weak.

But he wanted us to know he wasn't going to be bossed around. He had finally read the documents we sent him, Freeman's notes from his meetings with Lou, and he wasn't too happy about what he had read.

"It's inaccurate," he said. "There are things that are left out. Some of what's left out is critical."

Dave explained that the microphones weren't set up yet. My dad didn't care.

"I'd rather talk about things before we get into it," he said. "I don't know what's going to be covered. I'm very proud of some of the things I've done in my life!"

Dave told him we could talk about a few things before the tape got going. He said my dad ought to be proud of his son. "Howard has been interviewing all these people," he said. "Doctors, patients, psychiatrists . . . He's the worldwide expert on this thing now."

My dad wasn't going to listen to anyone tell him to be proud of his son. And he wasn't going to miss an opportunity to knock me down to size, either.

"I've always been proud of my son, even when he was not exactly the *sweetest* kid in the world," my father said. "Howard puts his pants on one leg at a time like everybody else, but he's a fine boy."

When the mikes were ready, Dave told me we could get started. My dad said, "Okay. Fire away."

Just like before, his answers were evasive. He had a sort of impatient, sarcastic manner, like he was lecturing a group of not very bright students.

He insisted that Lou had never told him half the things she told Freeman. He said he didn't think there was anything really wrong with my behavior or with me. "I did not see the things she was describing," he said. "I never did see them. I saw a normal boy that was not getting the affection he got before."

In fact, the problem, as he saw it, was that I had been given *too much* affection as a child. My real mother had spoiled me. She gave me all her attention, leaving none for her husband or her other son. Then, when he married Lou, I got a stepmother who had no affection for me at all. She was involved in a bitter ongoing dispute with her ex-husband. She was afraid of losing her children. If she had to sacrifice me to save them, so be it.

So, in his mind, the blame fell on my mother for loving me too much, on Lou for not loving me enough and for not telling him the truth about what was going on in the home, and on me for being defiant. *He* was blameless.

I tried something different. I asked him whether the operation had changed me. He didn't think it had. I asked him whether I might have ended up differently if I hadn't had the operation. He thought I would have ended up about the same. I asked him whether he regretted anything he had done with me, or if there was anything he now wished that he had done differently.

He said he didn't like to think about things like that. "If I were to sit and glower and dig over Lou and the things she did wrong, at the expense of the things she did right, it wouldn't *improve* me," he said. "It would damage my perception of what I should *become.*"

He explained that because of his mother's background in Christian Science, he didn't like thinking negative thoughts. He said my unhealthy obsession with my past wasn't going to help me with my present, or my future.

"It's over," he said. "I've got to live today, and you have to live today. What I'm trying to hope for is that you see the kind of person you *are,* not the person that other people perceive you to be, but what you always *have* been and what you always *will* be."

I didn't know what to say to that, but he liked that answer a lot. He said to Dave and Piya, "That's good! Put a star by that one!"

He answered some more questions, criticizing Freeman and the notes he took. He particularly objected to Lou's statements that he was violent, that he lost his temper and was "vicious" with me.

"I was reasonably fair with you," he said. "I won't say it was perfect. I wasn't perfect. Never will be. But I think the only thing I ever used on you was a shingle, wasn't it?"

I reminded him about the boards, about me having to choose the boards that he spanked me with. If the board broke, and he felt you needed some more whacks, he'd use his hand—which didn't break, unfortunately, and hurt like hell.

He didn't remember that, either. "I don't recall ever leaving you with a bruise on you or anything," he said. "Or where you couldn't sit down."

Dave was getting frustrated. He began asking questions himself. He asked my father again why he let Freeman go forward with the operation.

My dad said it was because Lou insisted. He didn't know what other choice he had. "The only option I would have had is to take Howard and Brian and move, and divorce her."

Dave asked why Lou hated me so much.

"I have no idea," he said. "You'd have to ask her—and she's dead."

I asked whether it was because I was so big. Was Lou afraid of me?

"I'm not a psychologist," he said. "I won't even try to play the game of what-did-it-mean."

We were getting nowhere. Dave passed me a note, and told me to show my dad the pictures of my operation again. We had to get a better reaction. So I pulled out the pictures and asked him, "Can I show you some pictures of the operation? Did I show you this picture already?"

"I never saw this picture before," he said. "God, you were a nice-looking boy! But your mouth is wide open—a Dully characteristic."

Urged on by Dave, I asked him, "Have you felt ashamed of me, ever?"

The silence that followed was incredible. He seemed to think about it forever. Then he said, "It's extremely difficult to answer. Because I don't carry those things around with me that way. I'm frustrated, you see. If I was ashamed of you, I'd be ashamed of me, because you're half me."

That wasn't exactly the no I was looking for. Dave urged me to go to the next question. Reading from my notes, I said, "I have a question that I'm not sure how to ask. Do you think that I'm owed an apology?"

"No," my dad said right away. "Because it serves absolutely no purpose. There is absolutely nothing to be gained by holding a grudge. If you wish to be issued an apology, well, it would be the equivalent of saying, 'Lou, say you're sorry you did it.' And I can hear her say, 'Yeah—when hell freezes over!' "

Dave stepped in again. He tried to get some kind of response. He asked what Lou thought would happen after the operation. He asked whether Lou was really trying to have me killed.

"I don't think she gave a damn," my dad said. "She just wanted him out of her life. That doesn't mean you're going to kill somebody. She made mistakes. She had strengths, too. But I never saw her as that type of person. No."

He sounded like he wanted to defend her—and to excuse himself for not knowing what she was up to.

"It's very difficult," he said. "This person you loved, and they were cruel, well, you just don't *do* that. Anybody who lives with someone who is cruel is *stupid.* And I didn't think I was stupid. I was color-blind. I didn't see."

Dave wasn't satisfied with that. So he showed my dad the pictures of me in the operating room again, and demanded an answer.

"Does it hurt you to see those ice picks in his eyes?"

That question made my dad angry. "Do you want me in the hospital—sick, lame, or lazy?" he barked. "Because what you're doing is asking me to dwell on something unpleasant and painful. And why should I? Looking at it will do what?"

My father was innocent. He was blameless. And now he was the victim. Never mind what had happened to me, and how he had contributed to it. Now *we* were hurting *him.* We were asking *him* to look at something painful in *his* life.

There was one other thing I needed to know. I asked him about my little brother Bruce. I told him about Lou telling Freeman that I had hurt him.

"No," he said. "That was a lie."

He remembered that it happened shortly after my mother died. We were living with my uncle Kenny. On this particular day, I wasn't even there. He had taken me up to Oakland, to the Chapel of Memories cemetery, to see where my mother's ashes were interred.

Bruce and Brian stayed at Uncle Kenny's, being watched over by Kenny's wife, Twila, and her two sisters. At one point, my dad said, one of the kids jumped into the playpen with Bruce and got rough.

"He started bouncing on the baby, and broke every rib in his body," my dad said. "When we came home, he was like a little bag of bones. It shook the daylights out of me."

There it was, at last. I knew I had not hurt Bruce. But it was still a relief to hear it from my own father.

Dave had one more question he needed me to ask my father.

I didn't want to. I asked anyway: "Here's an easier question: Do you love me?"

"Oh!" he said, then took his time answering. "This one is probably one of the greatest feelings a man has—when he sees his son for the first time. This is my flesh and blood, my contribution to mankind. And you were a cute little rascal, as far as I was concerned."

He couldn't answer the question. He couldn't say "I love you." He couldn't even say "Yes."

It was the last question I asked. My dad started complaining that he didn't feel well. He reminded us that we had agreed to quit if he wasn't feeling strong enough. Now he had some pain in his side and he wanted to go.

As we all got up to leave, there was some joking. Dave asked if I could give my dad a hug. I said I could if he was able to stand up. My dad said, "Does anyone here have a shovel?" and laughed. Dave and Piya began to pack up the microphones and recording equipment.

This was as close as I'd ever been to my father. I tried, one more time, to make a connection. The tape was still running. As we were getting ready to leave, I said, "I do want to thank you."

"I know it."

"I love you a lot. I—"

"Well, I think you're—"

"I want to say—I love you very much for this."

"And I *appreciate* that," he said. "I hope you're reassured about how you ended up—not about the problems you went through, but my perception of how you are *now*."

"I appreciate that."

As we were leaving, he surprised me. He said, "I think we had a good talk."

I told him I wondered why I had been so afraid to ask him these questions.

"You were probably afraid of my becoming irritated and easing away from you," he said. "You do not know your father! He does *not* walk away."

When I drove him home, he didn't seem angry. He didn't seem displeased with me. He was quiet. I took him back to his apartment and said good-bye.

That was April 2005. Dave and Piya went back to Brooklyn. There was nothing for me to do but wait.

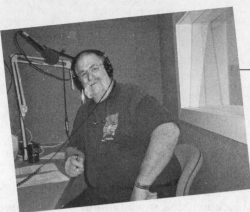

Chapter 16

Broadcast

L ife returned to normal for me and Barbara. I was driving buses for Durham. We were living in Aptos. Through that winter and into the spring we were just waiting. We didn't know when the program would be broadcast. Spring? Summer? We didn't know.

Sometime in late winter I started recording the parts of the program that would stitch it together. I'd drive up with Barbara or sometimes my son Rodney, and we'd meet an engineer named Larry Blood at KUSP, the National Public Radio affiliate in Santa Cruz.

It seemed to take forever. I have a good voice for radio, or people tell me I do, but I don't have radio-perfect diction. It took me quite a few takes to get some of the lines right. We'd have to tape them over and over.

For example, Dave and Piya had interviewed a woman named Angelene Forester, whose mother received the first transorbital lobotomy that Walter Freeman ever performed in his Washington, D.C., office. We had tape of Angelene talking with her mother.

"He was just a great man," her mother said.

"As a child, you kind of see into people's souls," her daughter agreed. "And he was good, at least then."

It was a powerful piece of tape. The problem was the mother's name. It was Sally Ellen Ionesco. Sally-Ellen-EYE-OH-NESS-CO.

I don't know about you, but for me that's hard to say. The script called for me to say, "His patient was a housewife named Sally

Ellen Ionesco." I stumbled over it so many times that we rewrote the line. In the broadcast, I just referred to her as "Ellen Ionesco," without the "Sally" part.

In May 2005 Barb and I moved house. I had recently cashed in my 401(k) plan from driving buses. I had enough money to buy my own place. We found a spot in a mobile-home community designed for seniors. I was barely old enough. Barb wasn't nearly old enough. But it was a good location, and it was affordable. For the first time in my life, I was living in my own home. That felt great.

Waiting for the radio broadcast to take place wasn't great. It seemed like it took forever. Finally, we were told it would air in November.

In advance of that, I met a few reporters. I met a whole crew from *People* magazine. They came up to San Jose to meet with us. They bought me a wardrobe for the photo shoot. They said they wanted me to look nice for the pictures. I could have looked nice wearing things out of my own closet, but I wasn't going to say no to some new clothes. We went down to the beach in Santa Cruz. They took pictures of me wearing tan slacks and a brown Pendleton-style shirt.

Then it was time for the main event.

Once again, I refused to fly. We arranged tickets for the train. Barbara couldn't get off work. So I took my son Rodney. We had a nice ride across the country. Then, Barb's schedule changed and she was able to join us. Rodney and I arrived in New York and got picked up by a Sound Portraits person at Penn Station right around the same time that someone else from Sound Portraits was picking up Barbara at JFK.

The broadcast was scheduled for Wednesday, November 14, 2005. The premiere was scheduled for the Monday before. It would be held at Bellevue, the famous New York mental hospital. The reception would be in the hospital library.

I knew all about Bellevue. Any person my age did, from cartoons and TV shows of the fifties and sixties. That's the place
where they took the crazy people. And that's where they took us
that Monday night.

It was almost empty when we arrived. I thought maybe no one
was going to show up. Then people started coming in. I couldn't
believe how many of them came. There were two hundred people,
plus a lot of press. There were people from CNN and the *New York
Times*.

It looked like a cocktail party. People were standing around,
chatting. But it was kind of weird, because a lot of them were chatting about *me*. That was a new thing. People were looking at me.
People were nodding at me, like they knew me.

They sat me and Barbara and Rodney down right in the
front row. Some of the other people from the broadcast were there,
too, like Carol Noell, Freeman's colleague Dr. Lichtenstein, and
Freeman's biographer, Jack El-Hai.

I was nervous. I felt like I was baring my soul. Everything about
me was going to be out there, for the whole world to see and hear.
What would that be like? I had kept these things secret from most
of the people I knew for almost my whole life. As far back as Agnews and Rancho Linda, I never told anyone about my lobotomy.
Now I was doing a national radio broadcast that was *called* "My
Lobotomy."

The program ran twenty-two minutes. It was very serious, very
somber. It began with voices I didn't know. And music. It was very
sad music—a piano playing something soft and sad underneath
these voices—that I found out later was written by Philip Glass.
The voices were talking about Freeman, and his lobotomy.

"We went into a room and there was a stretcher there . . ."

"He came in with something of a flourish, and he had his
valise . . ."

"And the first person was brought in and strapped down, and
given an electroshock."

"He had an instrument . . ."

"It was an ice pick."

"And then he'd shove it up into the forward part of the brain . . ."

"There was total silence among those of us who were watching. It was riveting."

There was total silence in the Bellevue Hospital library, too. You could feel the heaviness in the air. Then—the voice of Dr. Freeman, from an old, scratchy recording: "This is Walter Freeman, M.D., Ph.D. I am seventy-two years old now. . . ."

And then, not scratchy and old, but sounding like I was right there in the room, it was me.

"This is Howard Dully. In 1960, when I was twelve, I was lobotomized by this man, Dr. Walter Freeman. Until this moment I haven't shared this fact with anyone, except my wife and a few close friends. Now, I'm sharing it with you. . . ."

The audience heard me interview Frank Freeman. He remembered a drawer in the house where his father kept several ice picks. "A humble ice pick!" he says.

He has an aw-shucks sort of personality. He says things like "Good heavens!" He says it was "a darn good experience" to finally meet one of his father's patients.

He doesn't seem too concerned when I tell him I'd been lobotomized at the age of twelve. Then I ask him if he's proud of his father.

"Oh, yes," Frank says. "He was terrific. He was really quite a remarkable pioneer lobotomist. I wish he could have gotten further."

Other interviews follow. There's Angelene Forester and her mother, Sally Ellen Ionesco. Then comes Dr. Elliot S. Valenstein, author of *Great and Desperate Cures,* the history of brain surgery. He gives some historical context for the invention of the transorbital lobotomy, and tries to explain how such a brutal operation became so popular.

Next is the interview with Carol Noell. You hear us being introduced, shaking hands. You hear Carol describing her mother, who'd been operated on when Carol was just a little girl.

"Isn't she pretty?" Carol says. "She was so smart. . . ."

During this part of the program, sitting in the dark in the Belle-vue library, Carol took my hand, and held it tight for the rest of the show. She was obviously upset. She needed someone to lean on. Barb was a little bothered by this. But it didn't mean anything. Carol just needed someone to hold on to right then.

The conversation on the tape gets emotional. You can hear Carol's voice breaking. It's hard for her to talk about. She asks me why we're stirring up these painful things that happened so long ago and can never be corrected.

"How come it is that we're at the age we are and we can't seem to say, 'Okay, that was then, this is now'?"

"Because it's not okay," I tell her. "It's not finished."

The sad piano music comes back up. Then it's Dr. J. Lawrence Pool.

"I am now ninety-seven years old," he says. "I dedicated my life to brain surgery. I did not approve of Dr. Freeman's ice-pick method—no. I tell you, it gave me a sense of horror."

Then the audience heard me going to the George Washington University archives. "My file has everything," my voice on the tape says. "A photo of me with the ice picks in my eyes, medical bills. But all I care about are the notes. I want to understand why this was done to me."

First, I read out loud from Freeman's notes: " 'Mrs. Dully came in to talk about her stepson who is now twelve years old.' " Then I speak: "It's pretty much as I suspected. My real mother died of can-cer when I was five. My dad remarried, and his new wife, my step-mother, hated me. I never understood why, but it was clear she'd do anything to get rid of me."

There were more sections of the notes, the buildup from Lou's first meeting with Freeman to that terrible entry on December 3, 1960: " 'Mr. and Mrs. Dully have apparently decided to have Howard operated on. I suggested they not tell Howard anything about it.' "

There was total silence in the Bellevue Hospital library. On the tape, there is only the sound of my voice, recorded as I sat reading Freeman's notes, finding out for the first time what really happened to me, and why.

" 'December 17, 1960: I performed transorbital lobotomy.' "

" 'January 4, 1961: I told Howard what I'd done to him today and he took it without a quiver. He sits quietly, grinning most of the time and offering nothing.' "

You can hear, on the tape, how hard this is for me. I say, "And I was supposed to fight all this? No way. How is a twelve-year-old kid supposed to stand up to something like this? It just wasn't fair. . . ."

I didn't know what Piya and Dave had done with that part of the tape they had on me from the archives. At the time, I'd broken down and cried. On the tape, I exhale heavily. Then the music comes back up. Now it is a lone violin, sorry and sad, joined by a string quartet.

The sound of my voice returns: "When my stepmother saw the operation didn't turn me into a vegetable, she got me out of the house. I was made a ward of the state. It took me years to get my life together. Through it all I've been haunted by questions. Did I do something to deserve this? Can I ever be normal? And, most of all: Why did my dad let this happen? In forty-four years, we've never discussed it once—not even after my stepmother died. It took me a year of working on this project before I even got up the courage to write him a letter."

The sound changes again. My voice changes again. You hear me say, "I'm here with my dad. I've waited for over forty years for this moment. Thank you for being here with me."

It's almost impossible for me to say this on the tape. You can hear how difficult it is. My voice breaks several times. At the moment, it was incredibly emotional. Piya and Dave recorded it just as it happened. I was almost overcome with feeling. You can hear that on the tape.

And you can hear how, for my dad, it's not emotional at all. He says, "I'll tell you anything that needs to be answered," like he was taking a test at the Department of Motor Vehicles.

I ask him, "How did you find Dr. Freeman?"

"I didn't," he says quickly. "She did. She took you."

I push him a little. "My question would be, naturally, why would you let it happen to me, if that was the case?"

He says he doesn't dwell on the "negative."

I push harder still. You can hear on the tape how difficult it is for me. "But this was, this has really affected my whole *life*."

"Nobody is perfect," he says back at me. "Could I do it over again? Would I have? Oh, hindsight's beautiful. Fifty years later, can I say this was a mistake? So was World War One a mistake!"

You could almost hear the audience turn against him. There was a gasp or two. There was some mumbling. The energy in the room changed. It was as if he had admitted everything. It was all out in the open now. This was the guy who had let me down.

But the tape doesn't attack him. What comes next is maybe the most powerful moment in the whole program.

"Although he refuses to take any responsibility, just sitting here with my dad and getting to ask him questions about my lobotomy is the happiest moment of my life," my narrator voice says.

Then you hear my voice change, and it's clear I'm talking with my dad again.

"I want to thank you for doing this with me. I never thought this would ever happen."

"Well, you see?" my dad says, all chirpy and cheerful. "Miracles occur!"

"Actually what I wanted to do was tell you that I love you. . . ."

"Whatever made you think I didn't know that?" he says. "You shaped up pretty good!"

". . . and I feel very happy about that."

"That's what I wanted to hear!"

The piano music comes up again. Even now, it's almost impossible for me to listen to that moment without crying. It's heartbreaking.

I'm opening up everything to him. I'm telling him I love him. I'm almost begging him to say he loves me, too. And he doesn't.

The narration continues. "After twenty-five hundred operations, Walter Freeman performed his final ice-pick lobotomy on a housewife named Helen Mortenson in February 1967. She died of a brain hemorrhage, and Freeman's career was finally over. . . ."

The last interview is with Rebecca Welch, from the day she and her husband took us to meet her mother, Anita McGee. Rebecca begins to cry when she asks me, "Do you know how many people . . . can't do what you're doing, and you're doing it for them?"

The section ends with the sound of Rebecca and her mother singing "You Are My Sunshine."

Then my voice returns.

> After two years of searching, my journey is finally over. I'll never know what I lost in those ten minutes with Dr. Freeman and his ice pick. By some miracle, it didn't turn me into a zombie, or crush my spirit, or kill me.
>
> But it did affect me. Deeply. Walter Freeman's operation was supposed to relieve suffering. In my case, it did just the opposite. Ever since my lobotomy I've felt like a freak—ashamed. But sitting in the room with Rebecca Welch and her mom, I know that my suffering is over.
>
> I know my lobotomy didn't touch my soul. For the first time, I feel no shame. I am, at last, at peace.

The end credits come on, with that piano music again. Then the program ends.

There was total silence in the room. The audience seemed to be in shock. Then they began to applaud. There was a lot of applause.

Dave Isay got up and made some remarks, and then introduced me and a few other people who were going to take questions from the audience. I was in a kind of daze. I was overwhelmed. And I was scared. The program had been very emotional for me. I had never heard it with the music in. I'd also never been in a crowd like this, with all eyes on me. And all of those people were applauding me. It was very powerful. And now I was going to have to answer questions from the audience, or maybe even the press.

Most of them were more like comments than questions. People wanted to talk about how the program made them feel. It was easy. I was afraid we'd get some hostile remarks, or hostile questions.

There was only one. Some person insinuated there was something dishonest about the way the show was written—that I was obviously not smart enough to have written my own lines, and that I didn't talk the way they made me talk on the broadcast. A person with a lobotomy couldn't be that creative or that artistic.

That wasn't true, but it was upsetting to hear someone say it. What did they know about what I was capable of saying or writing?

Luckily Dave took the question. He said that the whole program was a collaboration, and that many people had contributed to every aspect of it.

In fact, I think every word I say in the broadcast is something I had a hand in writing, or at least in choosing the words. I didn't do the research on Dr. Freeman's early experiments with prefrontal lobotomy. I'm not a scientist, or a historian. But I helped write the words I would say about that, once I had the information.

The following day we traveled down to Washington, D.C. It was the first time I'd been there since we got my archives. It wasn't snowy now. The city looked different. We rested in the hotel, and waited for the broadcast.

I called my dad to tell him the broadcast was scheduled for that Wednesday. All he said was, "Oh, okay. Good luck."

Later on, I had a call from my younger brother Brian. It was pure coincidence. I hadn't heard from him in a long, long time. He was calling to say he had some pictures to send me, pictures from our childhood that he had come across in his house.

I thanked him and said, "You know where I am, don't you?"

He said he didn't.

"I'm in Washington. They're about to broadcast my story on NPR."

He said he'd listen.

We went over to the NPR studio for the actual broadcast. I sat in the control room with Dave, Piya, Barbara, and Rodney. We listened. There were lots of high-fives when the program ended. There was a feeling of exhilaration, and of relief. It was over, finally. It had happened.

But it wasn't over. After the show, Dave and Piya and the rest of us were standing around on the street outside the studio. We had given up our badges and IDs, and were getting ready to go back to the hotel. Someone came running down and said, "We crashed the server!"

There were so many e-mails coming in, so fast, that the National Public Radio Internet server collapsed under the weight of them. They had something like four thousand e-mails come in all at once, just at the end of the show. Dave said that the Sound Portraits server had crashed, too. Since it was a small one, that was no big deal. But the NPR server crashing—that was a huge deal. The NPR server had never before crashed in its history, someone told us. They had more e-mail on the lobotomy story than on anything they'd ever done.

Because of that response, someone quickly organized a show for the next day. I was scheduled as a guest on the NPR call-in radio show called *Talk of the Nation*. Dr. Valenstein was also on, by telephone, from his home. We took calls from people who wanted to talk about lobotomy, or share their opinions, or ask questions. The most common question was "How could this happen?"

We stayed that night in Washington. Barb flew home the next day. Then Rodney and I got on the train and began the long ride home.

My father never really told me what he thought of the broadcast. Neither did Brian. I know they both heard it. Brian didn't have anything to say about it. My father's only remark was that they had taken his comments out of context. He didn't say he was angry, and he didn't say he was unhappy with the way it came out. The comment about World War I, he said, wasn't fair.

By the time I got back to San Jose, the reader e-mails were being forwarded to me. Someone from NPR printed out a whole batch and sent them to me. It was overwhelming. A lot of it was applause for the documentary itself.

"Yesterday's show must go down as one of the greatest and most moving pieces I have ever heard on the radio," one listener wrote. "That is the most powerful piece I have ever heard on radio," another said. There were lots of letters like that.

A lot of other writers said they had never written to NPR before. "I have been a dedicated listener for more than 25 years, but in all that time, I have never taken a moment to write to you about any story," one woman said. Another person said, "After 25 years of listening [to NPR] and never writing to express how many stories have deeply affected me, I have to say that 'My Lobotomy' may be the finest piece of storytelling I have ever heard."

Some of the letters were from physicians. One of them said, "As a doctor I find it sad that lobotomy was welcomed by 'traditional' medicine. . . . I know we must always watch out for 'quacks,' however most people do not realize that many of the most dangerous, outrageous therapies are the ones approved by the 'traditional' medical establishment."

A lot of other letters were written by people who identified with how I felt and how I was treated as a boy. Some of them said they were lucky not to have had a lobotomy themselves. "As a person who suffers from depression and anxiety, I might have been a patient of Dr. Freeman," one listener wrote.

In many of the letters, people talked about crying during the broadcast. They said they cried in their kitchens, in their cars, caught in traffic, or in their offices. One man said he had to fight back tears while he was working out at the gym. Another said that she and her two children were *all* crying. One man said he had listened to the story twice. "Cried both times," he wrote. "Will most likely listen to the story again online. Will cry, again."

Almost all of the letters talked about how honest I was, how brave I had been, what courage I had, or what a hero I was. (A lot of them also said I had a "wonderful radio voice," and several urged NPR to hire me as a full-time correspondent. Memo to NPR: I am still available.) Many of them wanted to commend me personally for having survived my journey. I was really surprised by how people wanted to congratulate me for doing what I had to do to survive.

To my amazement, I got a letter from a woman named Nancy Greene, who said she had worked in the Santa Clara County Probation Department at the time I was made a ward of the court and sent to Agnews. "I am so happy you have a good life," she wrote. She said that she was sorry about what happened to me, and that she'd do anything she could to help me put together the "puzzle pieces" of my life.

Even more surprising, I got a letter from Linda Pickering, the daughter of Lou's sister Virginia. She's the one who, according to her mother, said I gave her "the creeps." She wrote to tell me how moved she was by the broadcast. She must have seen *People*, too.

"I want you to know how happy I am for you," she wrote. "You are truly a miracle. I was only 17 when this travesty happened to you. All I remember is the face of a lost little boy. I remember that my parents were dead set against this happening to you, and I know they told my Aunt Lou exactly how they felt. It was the wrong thing to do."

Linda went on to congratulate me for what I had made of my life, against the odds. "You have turned out to be a very successful citizen, good husband and great commercial bus driver," she wrote. "Handsome, too!"

In her letter, she put in a kind word for Lou. "I do want you to know that [Lou] didn't stay the way she was in those days. People mellow as they age. They also want to atone for all the wrong things that they did during their lives. I have to believe that she regretted what she did to you before she died. She became a soft-spoken, gentle woman. You have a wonderful gift of compassion and forgiveness, and I hope that you can forgive her."

Wow.

I had said in the radio broadcast that, sitting with Rebecca Welch, I was at last at peace. I felt a lot more of that reading those letters. I had sometimes been bothered by ideas that I had during the recording and interviewing of the show that I was doing something wrong. Was I sensationalizing my tragedy? Was I cheapening it?

Back when he was trying to get me to agree to use my own name, to build the show around my experience, and to interview my father, Dave Isay had offered to make me a financial partner in the broadcast, and to share the earnings from the show with me.

Was I going to be criticized for making money off the misery I had experienced? Did I have the right to do that? It was my story, after all. It was my misery. I wasn't taking anything from anyone. I thought I was doing something noble.

The e-mails confirmed that for me. They made me feel noble again—not because I had these experiences and survived them, but because I came forward and told the truth about them, and, in doing that, helped people.

In the meantime, I went back to driving the bus for Durham.

Not long after the broadcast, I was contacted by some publishing people and asked to think about writing this book. I got excited about that. There were so many things that had to be left out of the radio show. We had recorded more than a hundred hours of tape, and we had only twenty-two minutes of radio time. This would be a chance to really get to the bottom of the whole story.

The book might also mean a little money. And I needed money. My son, Rodney, had lost his job, and he had to move in with me and Barb in our new place. Then my stepson, Justin, had similar problems. He was a husband now, and a father. So he and his wife and child moved in with us, too.

It's a one-bedroom, one-bathroom place. We were all over each other. No one had any privacy. I wished I had enough money to get an apartment for them. But I was having trouble keeping my own head above water. My cell phone got turned off, because I ran up such a huge bill on the train trip to New York and Washington and back and I couldn't afford to pay it. The bank was threatening to repossess my car. I had complaints from the people who ran our mobile-home park, saying that kids were not allowed to stay there, even as overnight visitors. If I didn't hurry up and find my sons a place to live, I was going to be looking for someplace to live myself.

That spring, I was invited to a high school reunion. The folks from Los Altos High School, who would have been my classmates if I had stayed in school, invited me to come to a Friday night party and a Saturday night reunion. After some hesitation, Barbara and I decided to go.

It was the right thing to do. I made a few contacts. I got to spend a little time with my brother George and his wife. I got to renew a few acquaintances with guys I knew in junior high school.

But when it was over, I felt left out. I felt left behind. I had nothing in common with these people. My life had been interrupted in ways they could never understand. Their lives had gone forward in ways that would never include me. I left the reunion feeling discouraged and alone.

Then something changed. I was offered a speaking engagement.

In the middle of the year I was contacted by someone representing the National Guardianship Association. This was a group of professional guardians, the people who are hired or appointed by the court to watch out for people who can't watch out for themselves. They were holding their annual conference in Newport Beach, California. One of them had heard the NPR show. They wanted me to come talk to their members.

I prepared a presentation for them, a package that combined the radio broadcast and a CD slideshow of pictures of me, Dr. Freeman, Lou, my dad, and so on. I made some notes on things I would want to say to people who worked as guardians. Mostly I wanted to tell them what happened to me, and how it might not have happened if someone had been looking out for my interests.

Barbara and I drove down. We stayed one night in Hollywood, and the next day drove to Newport and checked into the hotel.

The event was held in a huge ballroom. I was the keynote speaker. My talk would be the last event before the awards luncheon. It would be attended by all of the conference attendees. I got to the ballroom, and almost fainted when one of the conference aides told me the room was set up for four hundred people.

The room filled up. I tried not to look, or count how many people were sitting there. Then a woman with the NGA took the stage. She said, "We are now going to hear from Howard Dully, who has an extraordinary story to tell. When he was twelve years old, he was given a transorbital lobotomy. He spent the next forty years finding out why. Please help me welcome Howard Dully."

There was warm applause. Everyone watched the stage. But I didn't walk to the front of the room. Instead, I waited until the room got dark, then started the radio broadcast. As the sound of my voice filled the room, I started the CD. People could hear me saying "My name is Howard Dully" just as they were seeing a photo of me as a child.

The audience was very quiet. At certain points during the twenty-two-minute broadcast, they got even quieter. At the point when I'm reading from Freeman's archives and I say, "December 3, 1960: Mr. and Mrs. Dully have apparently decided to have Howard operated on," the room was totally still.

The radio broadcast ended. The lights came up. I walked to the stage. The applause thundered like a wave breaking over me. I was choked up. I was in tears by the time I got to the front of the room. So were several women in the front row. There was a lot of applause.

I talked for a few minutes, telling them some more details about my dad, Lou, Freeman, and the others. Then members of the audience had questions.

"Wasn't there any governmental control of lobotomies?" one man asked. "Was anyone ever *helped* by them?" another wanted to know. "How did you feel, mentally, after the operation?"

I answered as best I could. I said I also wondered about the authorities who might have protected me. I told them I thought some people had been helped by lobotomies, but far, far more had been hurt. I told them that after the operation I felt drunk, and not quite there. "I still feel, today, like I had one too many jolts of electroshock."

One person asked how I thought the lobotomy had affected my brain, and another wanted to know how it had affected my life. I said that I didn't know what had happened, organically, to my brain. "But I've had a terrible, disastrous life," I said. "Not because of the operation, but because of what happened *after*. I didn't learn how to live. It wasn't because I was a bad guy, or because society was wrong, but because I didn't know how to live."

I answered questions for about thirty minutes before the NGA hostess told the audience we needed to wrap up and move on to the awards luncheon. But there were still ten people holding their hands up, so I took a few more questions. One woman wanted to know how I got along with my father today. Another person wanted me to talk more about being locked up at Agnews. A couple of people didn't have questions at all—they just wanted to thank me for coming and telling my story.

"I want to thank *you*," I said. "I have spent a lot of my life trying to turn something that was very negative into something that's a little positive. Coming here, and talking to you—it helps *me*. Having the opportunity to talk to people about my lobotomy has made it possible for me to understand, at last, that there's really nothing wrong with me. I'm just human."

The NGA representative finally had to tell us to stop. The awards luncheon was scheduled to start, but all four hundred of her attendees were sitting and listening to me talk. So I thanked her, and thanked the audience, and we concluded. I was rushed at the stage by another ten or twenty people. I spent the next fifteen minutes being thanked by them, individually, for coming out and telling my story.

When it was over, walking toward the luncheon, holding Barbara's hand, I realized that I did feel, at last, truly at peace. I felt useful. I had found my place. I was no longer ashamed.

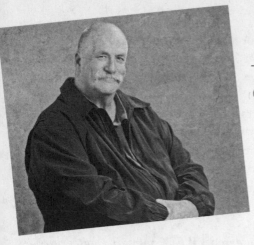

I am at the end of my journey now. I started wondering what was wrong with me more than forty years ago. I started asking what happened to me in 2000. Now I am finished.

The center of all the wondering and questioning was "Why me?" For a long, long time I was afraid that I had done something terrible. I was afraid I deserved what had been done to me.

Freeman's archives, and the research for this book, showed me that was wrong. My father, during the interviews, told me that was wrong. I now know that my stepmother had told Freeman lies. Freeman, more interested in performing the lobotomy than treating a patient, believed them.

When it was all over, I knew what had happened, and I knew how it had happened.

But I still didn't know why. Why did Lou hate me so much? Why did she and Freeman insist on lobotomizing me? Why was my father willing to go along with them?

My childhood was crazy. I feel like I grew up in a nuthouse. I had a crazy, scary stepmother, and for some reason I got the worst of her craziness. I wasn't locked in a closet, but I was systematically tortured, at least mentally. It was like I was trapped in some sort of play. My part was to always be in trouble. I was the bad guy who was always sent to his room.

Lou was mad. She was filled with anger and hate. But she

didn't hate her own son George, and she didn't hate my brother Brian, either. So it wasn't just a "stepmother problem." It seemed almost impossible not to believe there was something fundamentally wrong with me.

Was I crazy? I never *felt* crazy. But there must have been something wrong with me. Otherwise what they did makes no sense. This wasn't a secret operation they did on me. Dr. Freeman filled out forms. He wrote the words "transorbital lobotomy" on the hospital registration slips. He worked with radiologists and nurses. He was assisted in the operating room. He had signatures on the release papers from my father.

Many times I have wondered, *Where were the authorities?* Freeman wasn't a licensed psychiatrist. How could he determine on the basis of a couple of short office visits with me that I had been schizophrenic since the age of four? And why would anyone accept his diagnosis anyway without insisting that I be seen by someone with the proper training? Was there no medical standard for giving someone a lobotomy, especially a child? Is that all it took—one doctor saying it had to be done and he'd be the one to do it?

The sad thing is, the authorities were there. My family had been in contact with any number of doctors. I had been seen by, or Lou had consulted with, the Santa Clara County Family Services people, the experts in child mental health from Langley Porter, and the state mental health officers at Napa State Hospital. Some of them knew I was going to have a lobotomy. All of them knew Freeman was conducting lobotomies on children. Sometimes they protested after the fact, like they did the day Freeman took me and the other kids to Langley Porter to show us off. But why wasn't anyone taking steps to make sure Freeman wasn't operating on any more children? Why was this allowed to continue?

And has anything changed today? Where are the authorities now? How come any regular M.D. or pediatrician is allowed to diagnose depression or bipolar illness or ADD in children, and prescribe medications, without a second opinion? How many children are taking powerful brain medications now simply because their parents find them too difficult to handle? How many of those boys and girls are having their childhoods taken away from them, the way mine was taken away from me?

For a long time, the only answer I could find was that Lou and Freeman were right and I was wrong. If everyone knew what was happening to me and no one tried to stop it, it must have been the right thing to do. I must have deserved what they did to me.

But that's the biggest lie of all, bigger than any lie Lou told about me. It seems impossible to say that I was right and that my parents, my doctor, and the entire medical community around me were all wrong, but that's the ultimate truth. They were all wrong. To perform a transorbital lobotomy on a twelve-year-old boy was wrong. To perform it on a boy like me, who didn't even qualify by Freeman's published standards for the operation, was particularly wrong. But it would have been barbaric to do to any child.

Lou consulted with Dr. Freeman for two months. My father considered whether or not to do the surgery for only two days. The surgery itself took just ten minutes. But those ten minutes determined the next forty years of my life.

For most of that time, my life just passed me by. I felt like a failure. I felt like I never did what I should have done. I always fell back on the idea of "Poor me, I had the operation," instead of going out and getting a job and making my way in the world.

I became a victim—a full-time, permanent victim. My lobotomy was the explanation for everything that happened to me. My life didn't really start until I decided to go back to school and try to make something of myself. It started when I stopped acting like a victim.

What I see now is that we are all victims. The people who made the decisions that took away my life were victims, too, just like me. Freeman was the victim of distant, unloving parents, an unhappy marriage, and the tragic death of his son. Lou was the victim of a mother who abandoned her at birth, an alcoholic father, and an alcoholic first husband who left her with no money and two young boys to raise on her own. My father was the victim of his own father's early death, childhood poverty, the tragic death of his beloved wife, the tragic birth of and then injury to his third son, and the tragic decision to make Lou his second wife. He is as much the victim of my lobotomy, in some ways, as I am, just as they were all the victims of what was done to them.

That's true for everybody, I guess. We are all the victims of what is done to us. We can either use that as an excuse for failure, knowing that if we fail it isn't really our fault, or we can say, "I want something better than that, I deserve something better than that, and I'm going to try to make myself a life worth living."

Afterword to the Paperback Edition

My father died in the winter of 2008. He had been sick for much of the previous year, in and out of the hospital. His wife, Lois, had her hands full since she was also caring for her mother who was not doing too well. So Barbara and I spent a lot of time at my dad's house, taking him to his doctor's appointments, cleaning and cooking for him, and, on more than one occasion, rushing him to the emergency room.

My Lobotomy had been published several months earlier and even though I was nervous about it, I gave my dad and Lois a copy. But for a long time, I wasn't sure if they'd read it. I'd go over to their house to bring my dad some food or take him to see the doctor, and I'd see the book lying there. It had a bookmark in it. So someone was reading it, but I didn't know who and I was afraid to ask. I was afraid of what they thought about it.

My relationship with Dad was pretty much the same. He was short-tempered, and nothing we did was good enough for him. He didn't seem grateful that Barbara and I were there all the time, helping out. He didn't have anything nice to say about my son Rodney, either, even though he was around and helping out a lot, too.

Then, one day, I snapped. I said, "You know, you're not making this any easier. If you're going to criticize everything I do, I'm going to stop coming over here."

I think he was shocked. I was, too. It had taken me a long time to get to where I had some kind of decent relationship with my dad, and now maybe the book had ruined it.

Barbara and I left his house that day, and I thought, *Well, I guess I won't be going back over there.* But a couple of weeks later my dad called. He needed something. So I went over and did what I could to help.

It was hard to watch him being sick. He had always been strong and self-reliant. Now his legs were so swollen that he couldn't get out of bed, and he was so weak that he couldn't walk properly. He was still proud. He refused to get a walker. But it was obvious that he was fading fast.

I continued to wonder whether he had read my book. He never said, one way or the other. Lois had a few small things to say about it, mostly negative. But my dad never said a word. When I first told him about writing it, he wasn't very supportive. He said, "You know you'll never get it published." Then, when we got a publisher and had a contract, he said, "You'll never see a nickel of that money." Then he told me the reviewers would chew me up and spit me out. It turned out none of that was true. Book critics liked it a lot. We got dozens of really positive reviews. But, more important, *readers* liked the book a lot. I started getting tons of mail—letters, cards, and especially e-mails—from people all over the country who were deeply moved by what we had written.

The funny thing is almost none of them had any personal experience with lobotomy. I didn't get letters from other lobotomy victims, or children of lobotomy patients, or anything like that. But I got letter after letter from people who understood what it felt like to be twelve years old, unloved and misunderstood. They never experienced what I did, but they felt like I had felt. They wrote to thank me for expressing what they couldn't.

It was an exciting time. I did newspaper, magazine, radio, and television interviews. Journalists from Europe called me or came to my house to ask me questions. I was invited to take part in another

National Guardianship Association convention. Barbara and I took the train to Texas for that one, and had a great time checking out San Antonio.

The book money helped us make our life in San Jose a little nicer. Barbara and I were both able to pay off our car loans. We got new carpeting for the house, bought some new furniture, including a TV, and put in a new refrigerator and hot water heater. I bought myself a new laptop and a digital camera. I even rented an apartment for Rodney, Justin, and Justin's wife and baby.

When the book stuff quieted down a bit, I went back to work driving buses and teaching bus driving. Eventually I wound up back at Durham, teaching at Concord and then at their Hayward facility, before they finally moved me back to San Jose. Even then it was pretty stressful. I was teaching CPR and first aid, and driving special needs kids to school, while teaching bus driving in the classroom *and* doing behind-the-wheel instruction—all in one day.

Then, while we were busy worrying about my dad, Barb got sick. She had a series of small strokes and began to have trouble speaking. She would know what she wanted to say, but she just couldn't find the words to say it. She'd get tongue-tied, or would use the wrong words. She had trouble with numbers, too. She'd start to add two figures together, and all of a sudden they wouldn't make any sense to her.

It became clear that she would have to stop working soon. A large part of her job was writing reports, working with words and numbers. And, at least for now, she couldn't do that. I felt lucky that we'd made some money from the book, because it looked like we wouldn't be able to rely on her salary for a while.

Then she had an attack of what turned out to be Bell's palsy. Half of her face became paralyzed—not from the stroke, but from the Bell's. She started referring to it as her "ugly face." We made jokes about it, but it was hard for her. For the first time in her life, she felt defective, freakish.

Barbara being sick was hard for me. I was scared. Anything

involving the brain is obviously scary for me, not just because it's a delicate part of the body, but because of what doctors can potentially do to you up there.

Eventually she had to resign from her job. The doctors gave her exercises and medication for the stroke, and told us the Bell's palsy would just pass on its own.

In the spring of 2007, I made a little history: I became the first lobotomy patient ever to undergo a special type of MRI, a high-resolution MRI that could show exactly what Dr. Freeman and the lobotomy had done to me.

I had been contacted almost a year before by two scientists, one from Stanford University and one from the University of Southern California. They were leading a research study on the brain and had heard me on the radio. They decided it would be useful to meet me and take some MRI images of my brain for their study. We met for coffee at a Starbucks in San Jose. They told me what they wanted to do and I said that I'd be happy to help. I was excited about it. I was more than a little curious to find out exactly what had happened to me—the MRI would reveal that.

The two scientists were Bob Dougherty and Glenn Fox. Bob was a Stanford Ph.D. and the team leader. He was in his late thirties, a quiet guy with a beard and moustache. Glenn was his younger USC colleague. He was in his late twenties, and was more preppy and talkative.

They explained a little about their research. They were studying the brain and, in particular, its pathways. They were trying to figure out how certain parts of the brain talk to one another, how information travels back and forth on neural pathways between the different regions. One way to find this out is to look at what happens to people who have suffered brain trauma, such as a lobotomy.

Bob and Glenn were working with extremely powerful new MRI software, which was giving them brain images that were more detailed than anything seen before. They wanted to give me two different kinds of scans. The first was called a "high-resolution anatomical scan," that would give them very clear black-and-white images of the damage done. The second was called a "diffusion-weighted scan" that would create brightly colored 3-D images to reveal how the lobotomy had damaged the connecting tissue between the lobes of my brain.

In previous research experiments, they had done MRIs on control subjects and then given them "virtual lobotomies"—pretending, on a computer model, to cut into their brains with a pointer. They would try to predict exactly where Freeman's leucotome or orbitoclast instruments would have gone, and then which parts of the brain would have been damaged. After that they would try to guess what problems the person might have and what brain functions might have been lost.

But their experiments were mostly theoretical. They had never worked with an actual lobotomy patient. Even though there had been CT scans and even a few crude MRIs done many years before, no one had ever created these new diffusion images of a lobotomy patient's brain. And more important, they told me, no one had ever taken an MRI of a lobotomy patient who could be properly interviewed. Most of those patients were either dead or institutionalized. They couldn't tell their stories. But I could tell mine. I could tell the researchers what my life had been like before and after.

The way Glenn and Bob explained it, I was a special case in another way, too. Most lobotomy patients had experienced severe mental problems *before* their lobotomies. That's why they got them in the first place. They were either schizophrenic or severely depressed, meaning they had convulsions or fits, or were suicidal.

In my case, as far as anyone could tell, I was pretty close to normal before the surgery. So that gave Bob and Glenn a chance of seeing what impact a lobotomy had on a healthy human brain.

I was really excited about participating in the experiment. But it took a while to get it going. First Glenn and Bob had trouble finding an MRI lab that could run the new software they wanted to use. Then they couldn't find one in a place that was convenient for all of us—Bob was in Stanford, I was in San Jose, and Glenn was in Los Angeles. And when they did find one, there were still more problems. The machine wasn't big enough. My shoulders wouldn't fit through the opening and it turned out I was too heavy for the machine's drive gears. It was rated at 300 pounds, but I weighed about 350 at the time. When it came time for the machine to slide me into the MRI tube, it broke down.

Finally, in the fall, Bob and Glenn found a lab that had what they were looking for—an "open" MRI machine, a Siemens Magnetom Espree. It was powerful enough to get the high-resolution images they needed and large enough for me.

The machine was located at South County Imaging, in a little town called Freedom, just outside Santa Cruz. Because we were working with new software and a kind of MRI that had never been done before on a lobotomy patient, the people at the lab decided we'd need a whole day to take the images. They gave us a day when they figured no one else would be coming in for an MRI—November 21, the day before Thanksgiving.

Some time earlier I had been contacted by a news crew from England. They were making a documentary about medicine, a five-part series on the history of surgery. One part was about brain surgery, and lobotomy and Dr. Freeman. And a part of *that* was going to be about me. So they decided to film me, undergoing the MRI.

When the time finally came, it was a fine winter day—clear, bright, and cold. You could tell we were near Santa Cruz because there was one lone redwood tree in the lab's parking lot. All around us were fields, acres and acres of farmland and new tract homes.

There we met up with Bob and Glenn, and another colleague of theirs, a woman named Michal Ben-Shachar. Glenn took us inside and introduced us to Andrew Stafford, a cheerful guy with a goatee who would help them conduct the scans.

They were all really excited. I was, too, and nervous. All I could think about was what they would find. I'd heard jokes my whole life about having half a brain. I'd been called dummy, stupid, and brain-less. Is that what we were going to learn today—that all that was true?

I was afraid that something *else* might be wrong with me, too. What if I had a brain tumor or brain cancer? Or what if I had already had a stroke? I saw my life as a long series of catastrophes. Were there others I didn't know about? Was this going to be the next one?

I was prepared for the worst. But I was also aware that we were making history. I kept thinking that what we were doing would outlast me. I had written a book about my lobotomy. Now images of my brain were probably going to wind up in a textbook some-where. I liked that idea.

But the MRI took a long, long time to get started. First there was the machinery, and getting me positioned properly in this big round doughnut where the images would be taken. Then there was a lot of hubbub with the camera crew—figuring out where they could put the camera, where they could put the lights, where they could put their microphone. Every time it looked like we were ready to begin, there would be some technical glitch and we'd have to wait again.

Throughout the procedure, the host of the show was interview-ing Glenn, Bob, and Andrew and asking them questions like: What did they expect to see? Why was this experiment important? What was a lobotomy supposed to do? Was Freeman a visionary or a monster? From the other room, where I was waiting, flat on my back, I'd hear little snatches of the interview and wish they'd all hurry up.

At last they were ready. The door to the MRI room was shut. The large machine began to crackle and hum. If you've ever had an MRI, you know what I mean—it's incredibly loud and kind of scary. Glenn and Bob had given me earplugs to wear, but it was still weird.

And it took a long time, too. It took them more than an hour to take the pictures, while I lay there waiting, just waiting.

Finally they let me come out. They gave me a soda, and we all ate some sandwiches provided by the clinic.

Afterward Glenn and Bob explained what they had seen on the MRIs. They told me a bunch of times it was all premature, that it would take weeks or even months of study before they would really know what it all meant. But they could see certain things right from the start. They showed me an image of my brain.

At first, I was relieved. There it was! It looked pretty much like a normal brain. Like I said, I had been made fun of my whole life. My Dad had called me brainless, before the lobotomy *and* after. So seeing my brain in there, seeing it whole, just made me feel better.

Glenn and Bob were incredibly excited. They showed me exactly where the "icepick" instruments had entered. It was easy to see. There were these two dark areas, like tunnels, coming up from my eye sockets. They were dark, Glenn told me, because when brain cells are damaged, they die and are absorbed by the fluid in the brain, which fills up the empty space. They told me later that they hadn't known what to expect. They thought it was possible they wouldn't see much, or that what they saw wouldn't be clear enough to tell them anything. Instead, they had a perfect road map of the lobotomy that showed where the knives went in and the exact area of the brain they had damaged.

They also told me, much later, that the images surprised them in another way. Having met me, they didn't think the MRI would show them much actual damage from the lobotomy. Maybe the procedure had failed or maybe Freeman had had second thoughts and decided not to do it at all. They thought I seemed too normal to have had a lobotomy. They'd heard the radio broadcast. They'd heard about the book. They'd met me and Barbara, and hung out with us a little. They had some ideas about lobotomy patients, and I didn't fit the image.

Freeman's goal in conducting a lobotomy was to sever the pathways between the front lobes and the body of the brain. Freeman thought he could interrupt the bad feelings that caused depression, anxiety, and other mental problems. But when he did a lobotomy, he was severing all sorts of *other* pathways, too. Some of them involved vision, some involved language, and some seemed to involve emotion and logic.

Bob and Glenn had expected someone who had undergone a transorbital lobotomy to have real problems as a result. The typical Freeman patient, they said, would not have been able to hold down a job and would not have been able to sustain an extended personal or romantic relationship. He would probably have had difficulty controlling his emotions and he may even have been sociopathic.

When they met me, they were introduced to a happily married guy who had a job, two kids he supported, and also a father he helped care for. I had my own house and made my own car payments. I wasn't institutionalized or on psychiatric medications. I was too normal. So they were shocked, they said, when the first MRI pictures appeared on Andrew's computer that day. The pictures they saw were of a badly damaged brain.

I asked them later, if they only had the MRI to look at, what kind of patient would they have imagined? What would that patient be like?

"He would require permanent institutionalization," Glenn said. "He would not be able to care for himself. He would not be able to function in the world at all."

Wow. So *that's* why they got so excited about those first images.

I think Barb might have understood this before I did. She got really emotional, and had to leave the room several times. I could tell she'd been crying.

It took forever to do the MRI, transfer the MRI images to DVD, and to finish up all the interviews. It would take much longer, maybe months, before the images could all be properly analyzed. So for now, Barbara and I said good-bye to the British film crew, and to Glenn, Bob, and Andrew. We drove out to the coast, and down Highway 1 to a little fishing town called Moss Landing, where there's a great seafood restaurant that serves the best clam chowder in the world. We ate dinner before driving back to San Jose.

• • •

Life goes on.

A week after the MRI in Freedom, I celebrated my fifty-ninth birthday. I went back to work. Barbara slowly got better, but my dad slowly got worse. Then, one day, we got the call saying the end was near. I contacted my brothers and my uncle Kenny. I told them it didn't look like Dad was going to make it through the weekend. Everyone planned on arriving by Sunday morning, but he died that Saturday, before some of them could get there.

We set the memorial service for January 31. That morning, my brothers began arriving—Brian from Chicago, and George and Kirk from the Pacific Northwest. Cleon didn't come, but I didn't expect him to. When it was time for the service, we all got in our cars and drove to the Roller Hapgood and Tinney Funeral Home in Palo Alto.

My father had been involved in a lot of organizations, so there were a lot of people at the memorial. There were people who knew him from his years as a teacher, as a volunteer in the sheriff's department, and as a member of the National Guard. There were men and women in long white robes, and other outfits—my father had also been a Mason, a member of the Scottish Rites Temple, and of something called the Sovereign Military Order of the Temple of Jerusalem.

"Amazing Grace" was playing in the lobby of the funeral home. A big band version of "Don't Sit Under the Apple Tree (With Anyone Else But Me)" was playing inside the chapel. I sat in the front row, next to Lois and my brothers. About a hundred people sat in the rows behind us. A man I didn't know, dressed in Masonic robes, got up and said a few words about my dad. A little white-haired woman got up and sang a hymn about being raised up on eagles' wings. Another man, who looked like a minister, got up and talked about "a virtuous and well-spent life." The Mason came back and talked about how we would all meet again "in the celestial lodge above, to part no more."

Finally the family got to speak. My uncle Kenny went first. He told a story I had never heard about how my dad had saved him from drowning when he was a little boy. He broke down at the end, and said, "He was a character—and he was a great older brother."

I got up next and read a letter that had been sent to me by a retired superior court judge who had known my father when he worked as a bailiff. He had also had my father as his sixth grade elementary school teacher in 1956. He remembered him as being extremely gentle and kind.

Then Brian got up. He shared some nice memories of Dad, and said he wanted to recite the poem that represented him the best, which was "If" by Rudyard Kipling. "If you can keep your head, when all about you are losing theirs . . . You'll be a man, my son."

Kirk spoke after Brian. He said, "Dad was a lot of things, and busy was always one of them." He made people laugh.

The Masonic guy returned. He said, "The march for our comrade Rod has come to an end. Comrade Rod is now in the hands of our Heavenly Father." The ceremony ended with a color guard and "Taps" being played on a bugle.

The reception was held a few miles away in Mountain View, at a clubhouse on a golf course. We ate finger food and drank beer and wine. There were no more speeches, but after a while someone got out a camera and said, "Okay—all the brothers!" For the first time in almost fifty years, Brian, George, Kirk, and I stood together to have our picture taken. Brian and I stood in the back, because we were the tallest. Brian put his arm around my shoulder and I put my hand on George's. At that moment, we were just like any other brothers.

It felt like the end of something. My father was gone, but my brothers and I were together. It felt strange, because it was so unusual, but it also felt good.

A few months after that day in Freedom, I again heard from Bob and Glenn. They were working hard analyzing the MRIs.

They were shocked by what they were seeing, and by how difficult it was to reconcile the images with me. They were amazed by the story the images told of the human brain.

If Freeman had performed the same lobotomy on me as an adult, they said, I would have been a vegetable. That's how badly damaged my brain was. I wouldn't have been able to survive outside of an institution. I would have stayed at Agnews forever.

But my brain, when Freeman got to it, was young. It was still growing. After the surgery, it adapted to the lobotomy and found ways to compensate for it. The parts of my brain that Freeman hadn't damaged grew stronger. This was very unusual, according to Bob and Glenn, but not unheard of. Bob had read about a teenage girl in Germany who began to experience some weakness in her left leg and arm. Her parents took her to the doctor. The doctor referred them to a neurologist, who got worried—he discovered that she was weak on her entire left side. So he ordered an MRI, which showed that the girl, basically, had no brain on the right side. She had probably been born that way; the right hemisphere of her brain had just never developed.

In an adult, if the right hemisphere is destroyed or damaged that severely, forget it. That person would be finished. They would experience terrible problems with vision, language, reasoning . . . with everything.

But this girl's problem had begun at birth, or even in the womb. So her brain had adapted right from the start. The neurologist found that, other than some weakness on the left side of her body, she had no other problems. She was perfectly healthy and, even though she might not make it to the Olympics, she'd be able to play sports and do all the things that teenage girls do. She would be able to live a totally normal life.

I was a bit shaken up by that story, and by what Glenn and Bob said about the damage done to me. But then I started to see things a little differently. I had always thought it was horrible that I underwent a lobotomy at the age of twelve. How could anyone do something so barbaric to a child? I always felt sorry for myself because this terrible thing had been done to me when I was so young. But now I saw that I was actually fortunate to be young when it happened. If I'd had the same lobotomy even five years later, when I was seventeen, I might not have had a life at all.

Today, I count myself lucky. I'm lucky to have survived Freeman, and to have survived my childhood and the aftermath of the surgery. I've gone through a lot—institutionalization, homelessness, alcoholism, drug addiction, having a criminal record, and an overall sense of being unloved and unlovable.

But I don't feel those things today. I feel blessed. I feel happy and grateful that I have lived long enough to tell my story.

Acknowledgments

I could never have done this without the help of a large number of people. I am grateful to them all.

I would like to thank Christine Johnson, who started psychosurgery.org and introduced me to Dave Isay and Sound Portraits, and Carol Noell Duncanson, who introduced me to Christine.

I would like to thank Dave Isay and Piya Kochhar. Dave is a man who changes lives, and Piya is the world's greatest con artist. She got me to fly! And she got me to interview my father. I'm still not sure how she tricked me into doing those things, but I love her and Dave very much.

I would like to thank all the friends I made at National Public Radio, and at Sound Portraits. I'd like to particularly thank Larry Blood and the other people at KUSP.

I would like to thank all the people who agreed to be interviewed, particularly Frank Freeman and Dr. Robert Lichtenstein.

I would like to thank Dr. Elliot Valenstein for his book *Great and Desperate Cures,* and Jack El-Hai for his book *The Lobotomist.* These men and their writings were very helpful in the assembling of this book. Also very helpful to me were David Anderson, Lyle Slovick, and the other archivists at the Walter Freeman and James Watts Collection, Special Collections and University Archives, The Gelman Library, George Washington University.

For their help in setting up the MRI scans in Freedom, I would like to thank Bob Dougherty of Stanford University and Glenn Fox of the University of Southern California. Thank you also to Andrew Stafford and Becky Shoemaker of South County Imaging, for donating their time and facilities, and also Katia Moubarak, of Siemens Medical Solutions, for her assistance.

My family has been very patient with me through this ordeal. I want to thank my dad for putting up with my questions, and his wife, Lois, for watching over my dad. I love them both so much.

My sons, Rodney and Justin, were very helpful to me, too. I'm so proud of them both.

My brothers, George, Brian, and Kirk were also very patient with my questions. They were willing to go back to a painful place and time. I'm honored to be their brother. I'd like to thank my uncle Kenneth for helping, too.

I want to thank my agent, Gary Morris of the David Black Agency, for introducing me to my cowriter, Charles Fleming, and my editor, Heather Jackson. I want to thank Charles and Heather for believing in this project.

And, last, I want to thank Barbara Lee Dully, my wife and partner. She stuck by me when I was down in the dumps, and lifted me up, time and time again, by showing me that it was all going to work out someday. She was right. I love her, and am honored by knowing her.